VENEFICII GENERIBUS

BOOK OF SORCERY STYLES

Ambroze Hildreth

Published in the United States of America

ISBN 979-8-89395-962-8 (SC)
ISBN 979-8-89395-960-4 (HC)
ISBN 979-8-89395-961-1 (Ebook)

Library of Congress Control Number: 2025912809

Battle Mage Inc
145 W Broadway
Long Beach, CA 90802, USA
ambrozehildreth@outlook.com

Ordering Information and Rights Permission:

Quantity sales. Special discounts might be available on quantity purchases by corporations, associations, and others. For details, contact the publisher at the address above.

For Book Rights Adaptation and other Rights Permission.
Call us at toll-free 1-888-945-8513 or send us an email at
admin@stellarliterary.com.

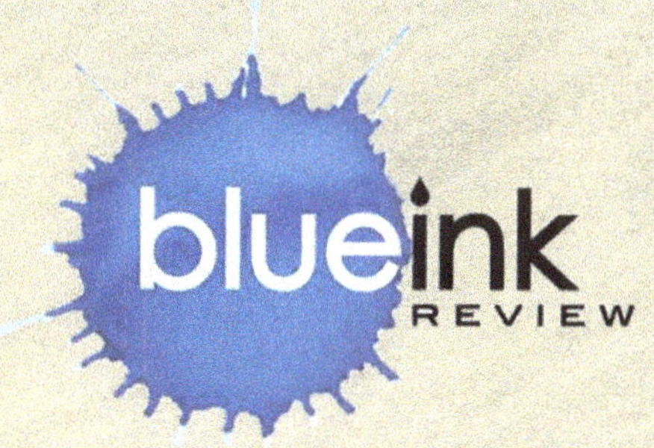

Veneficii Generibus: Book of Sorcery Styles
Ambroze Hildreth
Battle Mage, 204 pages, (paperback) $25.99, 9798893959628
(Reviewed: May 2025)

Ambroze Hildreth's self-described "scientific approach to performing the mystic arts" is an extensive compilation of spells grouped according to specific guidelines, preceded by a survey of the belief systems he utilizes.

Intended for those on the journey "to becoming a wizard," the book establishes basic laws that ground the practices, many of which "break some societal illusions." He defines science as "The subconscious of the universe...the order we follow, the law in which things work." Chemistry is "a number-like system that's naturally made"; biology is based on these chemical laws which also "creates our physics."

When describing human consciousness and evolution, Hildreth implies an underlying moral code rooted in individual actions: "[T]echnique, skill, and moments" create power, which "is earned... You are worthy of what you create yourself into." He also notes that "Your worst enemy and rival is yourself."

Hildreth provides some framework of understanding for those who wish to practice the book's spells. Chakras, auras, and processes, along with Chinese, Celtic, and Norse representations of the Seeds of Life, come into play, among other elements. The author also offers a series of "mind-understanding" tools, including meditation, "biofield manipulation," and third eye exercises.

Charts and illustrations complement the text, and readers can easily dip into the portions of the book that are personally relevant, rather than reading straight through.

The book is not for skeptics, however. The author's definition of science is based on his own belief system, and he assumes readers are onboard with his viewpoint. It's also not for beginners, as terms are often not defined and instruction can be extremely cursory ("Taste the feeling of an atom"; "Create a connection with the earth, feeling its charge, and its nanoteslas"). The author employs plentiful jargon that can be off-putting ("emomancer," "biomagnetism concentration," "subducti").

While clearer explanations would benefit all readers, those who seriously study the "do-no-harm" forms of magic and healing will find an abundance of ideas to investigate here.

Also available in hardcover and ebook.

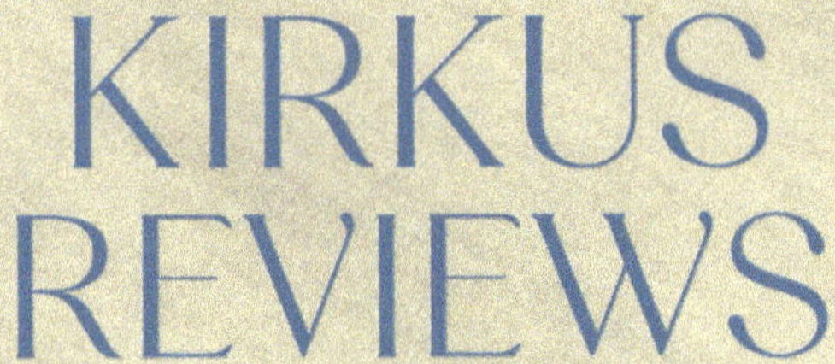

TITLE INFORMATION

VENEFICII GENERIBUS
Book of Sorcery Styles
Ambroze Hildreth
$25.99 paperback
ISBN: 9798893959628
April 10, 2024

BOOK REVIEW

A book of practical approaches to the personal and spiritual aspects of wizardry.

As Hildreth explains, this book is designed for readers to carve out their own paths to "becoming a wizard." (Wizardry, per the author, is about understanding and manipulating worlds both inside and outside of an individual.) First, Hildreth provides explanations of the basics: One must understand the nature of different numbers and colors. Take zero; it is "significant for nothing, and the most literal nothing is space." Colors also have meanings, such as green representing kindness and blue representing honesty. The author offers instructions on practices like meditation and prayer. Hildreth introduces techniques like "Mindscape Building," used to "allow the exploration of your inner mind and turn it into a valuable tool." With this tool sharpened, readers can access the mysteries at the heart of the book in chapters with titles like "Sound Mage," "Time Mage," and "Tree Mage." These tend to run to a page in length and are thick with information. In a chapter titled "Mirror Mancer," readers learn that they have access to something called the "mirror realm"; this is useful if one seeks to set mirror traps for "negative entities and demons." It's all a lot to take in. Even though the text includes fewer than 200 pages, it feels much longer as it incorporates a vast array of subjects that range from the different layers of existence to "using a micro-movement" to generate an echoing thunderclap. While the material can be intimidatingly abstruse, the book is written in serious, straightforward language that allows the reader to look at the world in a new way. Even if one does not set out to complete the path to practicing sorcery, it is easy to appreciate a statement like "We are an electrical system within ourselves, and with proper techniques, we can utilize and direct that power." The work ultimately provides a tangible starting point to processing information that is not always as mysterious as it may first appear.

A straightforward (if dense) guide to understanding one's inner, esoteric abilities.

EXCERPTING POLICIES

Outlook:

This is a spell book that helps organize ability into styles, allowing focus, cross-practice, and mastery of multiple schools. This book will allow the user to carve their path. This is a scientific approach to performing the mystic arts. Please keep an open mind and understand that the truth is always the best answer, regardless of what is given here. Intelligence is a practice.

This book is not built on situational truth, only scientific understanding. This is a take-it-or-leave-it teaching. Take what you can from this, and it will help you find your poetry. Be skeptical and you may miss the bigger picture. This is a condensed version of what takes years of training. Regardless, the whole point is to gain knowledge and always seek further training even beyond this book.

Each book is meant to be different. At the end of the book, there are pages for further study of spells, or cross-style spells. These pages are meant for you to fill in, making these books personal and part of your journey to becoming a wizard.

Contents

The Cleansing

First, we must understand some basic laws that allow further understanding and cleanses thought. You must read through this part to fully gain the benefits of magic, as well as understanding truth creates the best path to use the arts. This will break some societal illusions that have been created over the years.

Truth is not always easy and not always what we want to hear. Understand that truth is fact and is always there regardless of the point of view or opinion. Learn to seek and understand the truth even if it seems harsh. Disregarding truth is a path to denial. Listening to want and not need is also a path to denial. When we listen to want it can trap us in placebos. Placebos are easily defeated by listening to the truth. Be truthful to yourself, and then you are the truth.

The universe is based on truth. The most literal physical reality is the most possible reality, and so far, as we know, the only one. We can get caught in frequency and energy confusion, as well as dimensions and timelines confusion. Just know that sources of all energy are always from a source of matter. All matter is the source of all frequency, all energy, and all dimensions. All timelines also follow this law and do not exist without matter. If you find the source, you can fix the problem. Know your sources.

The subconscious of the universe is what we call science. It runs all things and allows all things to be, however it is not tangible. It is the order we follow, the law in which things work, and what allows us to be. It follows at the smallest of levels, all the way out. Science is the study of how we exist. We exist based on our matter, and our matter has a law, which is undying truth. In that study you will find that we react to a number-like system that is naturally made, we call that order chemistry. Our biology is based on these chemical laws. Chemical law creates our physics, for you need matter for physics to exist.

We must understand that we are mechanical and electrical by nature. Our DNA is the source of our being. We are made to be able to work off the subconscious. Understanding the subconscious is a state, however, it is the first state of all beings. Consciousness is a byproduct of living, and we gain memory by obtaining information through our senses. The brain is mostly involuntary which sustains us. It is through the involuntary that the voluntary can be created. The next step is storing memory, which is organized by how the information is obtained. We obtain information through sensory, reaction, and movement. This is how we react to the outside world. This is made possible based on the literal structure of the brain.

Listening is always first. The senses are based on listening, and further senses of our involuntary listening to our body's states, like hunger and thirst. We have internal senses, which are based on sleep, eating, drinking, and breathing, to external senses, which are touch, sight, hearing, taste, and smell. We also have advance senses which our governed by outside sources, such as time and gravity. Everything is made from molecules, making them react and act the way they do, this includes frequency. Bacon tastes like bacon for a reason and not like lemons, wood feels like wood, not like metal, we do not decide the world of sensory, it is made that way.

Remember to listen to the body's needs not its wants.

Consciousness is a secondary system, generated by the subconscious, which is DNA and set value structures. So, we are our matter, which generates energy. We are not energy, we generate it. The body creates the mind and the soul. The mind is a state of consciousness, and the soul is simply the journey and the experience our matter goes through. It is not a tangible thing, and yet it is your personal sensory (tangible) experience. Now that we understand that, we can add to our memory through knowledge and movement, to develop skill and technique.

Our brain has set values that tell you stuff like when you're cold, or hungry. The brain also tells us when we want or like something, and when we don't like something or find something dangerous. We add to these things as we gain experience. Learning allows us to add to the basis of our experience, to improve our experience, and to our chances of survival. Every moment adds to our experience, and moments with emotional responses tend to add to those experiences due to their intensity. We are creatures that can adapt due to our nurture.

You are part of evolution. We are given a set nature/nurture genetic disposition from our parents. Nurture allows us to evolve due to our experiences and the ability to learn from them. We continue to do so with every experience we have, creating individuality from our parents. There is evolution based on viewpoint and action, which is our nurture. Organization of our thoughts can also aid our mental evolution. Our physical evolution is based on muscle development, food patterns, and environmental exposure. The physical aspect of evolution is always within our genetic and mechanical structural parameters. Choose how to evolve and understand how and why. It is important to understand that evolution usually involves genetic growth. This form of evolution is based on the parameters we already exist within.

Power is created through technique, skill, and moments. No one just gains power, power is earned. Anything you earn, you are worthy of, because you earned it. The gift is life, never accept a gift of power, and always earn the right. You are unbeatable this way.

You are worthy of what you create yourself into. No one can take your actions away from you. Remember, we also develop karma in life. Make yourself worthy of yourself, and you will always be worthy.

Your worst enemy and rival is yourself. What other people might be is not your concern, it is what you created yourself which is the concern. Others can be used as a measurement, however, in this book, you will find your own unique experience, and that no two people are the same.

We are all made of the same things (the periodic table of elements), just in different patterns and orders. So, we are different, but the same. The order is what makes us unique, for the order can also be the sequence of experience. To truly understand our nature, we must understand the physical literal.

The physical literal of nothing is space itself. We can organize the universe into two things, nothing, and everything else. So, nothing, and something. Something is what creates anomalies in nothing. All matter is the anomaly, that is the anomaly of matter. Nature is made up of something. The rules of nothing is literal, it is not the something.

The nature of something at our conditions of matter on earth is in the order of the periodic table. This means all things are nature, even technology is nature, just matter organized in a specific way to do a specific job. There is a difference between organic nature and nature. Water and air are not organic, however, needed to sustain life. We are built to the conditions of the earth, however a byproduct of its conditions.

All things are made of electrons, protons, and neutrons, all things are something and not nothing and therefore all of something is nature.

Fate does not chain you down. Fate is a predicted path, and our movements are unpredictable. What is predicted is the stars and planets and where they are going. They are fated and we are fated by where it is going. We are free from fate. Remember nature is naturally free and wild.

In the entirety of the infinite universe, it creates conditions that create and support life. We are the result of the universe, meaning all this just for us to say why, and how. We are an energetic positive, created to generate our experience, this is the entirety of existence and the universe's result. The answer is to preserve and protect what takes millions of eons to make, life.

A sin is causing harm unto another. So those that harm life and take the experience away from someone are technically a sin. The aim should be to protect life, so if you know how to harm you know how to heal. Serve life and you never fail.

Life is complicated and opinionated, so a passive way to serve life is to serve the earth. The earth sustains us all with its magnetic sphere. Without the earth we would have no home. To sustain the earth is to sustain humanity.

Society is manmade, and therefore could be done in hundreds of different ways. Clear yourself of superstition and the opinion of the masses by taking a scientific perspective of life. Logic will allow you to make yourself something new without the opinions of society. Science will inevitably be able to answer all political perspectives, which will eventually end in a scientific compromise. The truth is that we exist, that's a natural positive. That makes our planet a precious gemstone in the universe.

Earth is a kingdom in the universe, and a kingdom is not one without subjects. This is a kingdom, which develops a magnetic sphere due to a specific amount of matter. We develop an electromagnetic field at our level, just with the blood pumping, and reacting with the brain, via the iron in the blood. The earth develops a similar field at a larger level which sustains plants like trees, which create oxygen for the rest of us.

Earth is like a god in the universe, due to its rarity. It is a kingdom, and a haven to live. However, earth and other planets have a system of beings who serve life. This system is a system of once-conscious beings who serve the greater universe, in turn, they serve life, which in turn is serving kingdoms. They were once people like you and me, which found a greater path to serve in the greater consciousness. If you meet these entities on your journey, they serve the universe in a positive way.

People have called them God; however, their power was as big as they are. We only affect the physical space around us, and we are as strong as our matter is. Therefore, Earth is much larger than any of us. Earth will not bother you; it is neutral, and only conscious beings will try to gain something from you, however subconscious beings, or super benevolent ghosts, may respond at different frequencies, usually in the medium. Sometimes they come in different forms, that work at a benevolent level, serving life and earth, and usually respond passively to those who listen. Proof of listening is meditation.

Negative entities, like demons, or evil ghosts, are usually beings rejected by the greater kingdom. Remember, all is nature, which means even evil is nature. The root of all evil is selfishness. There is no negative, it is simply a different direction or lack of something. This works from physics to the spiritual.

Remember that the spiritual is generated by the physical. We are our matter, then there is a release or a lack of energy when we die. Our matter is no more and we deaminate. Lack of internal movement equals death.

A possible truth of the death cycle is reincarnation. However, the path is natural and therefore passive, it happens on its own. We can program ourselves in death, for example, once we are nothing, we could be anything in the next life, for reincarnation is not sexist, not racist, and not limited to one species. To sustain life is to sustain reincarnation. To be only our matter and to end with our bodies, regardless of how, we are not produced anymore, for that which allows the experience is gone. Deamination in death is the literal physical. Life and death are abstract from one another, meaning they are not connected, yet they exist and usually are linear. They are abstract like light.

The aura is made from the matter yet not the matter, this is how light works. The light from the sun is not physical matter, however, a wavelength that is generated from it. Tachyon theory suggests that the bradyon (or sun's wavelength) causes light particles when entering a particle atmosphere, which are planets like earth. The moon does not have a particle atmosphere, which causes the wavelength to have a different effect on the matter due to a lack of gasses on it.

If you remember anything from this, remember that the conqueror is wisdom. The greatest of all things is wisdom, no matter if it is evil or if it is good. For example, evil genius would not jeopardize themselves by harming another, so they stay good or play within the law. Not everything evil is bad, like a hammer can be a tool or a weapon.

Fear is in the reality of the situation; it only exists where the situation existed. Worry is manifested in the mind, usually from retribution or threatening possibilities. If it is not there it cannot harm you, so don't fear it, listen to your instinct, or internal listening, which can recognize harmful situations at the time of. If you don't worry or fear, when the time comes that you need the response, it will do so correctly.

Most emotions are reactions, such as anger, joy, sadness, and even love. Love is the reaction between two people, and there are millions of combinations. but love isn't always associated with people, it can be associated non sexually, like with the earth, with your children, and or with animals. It is easy to attain if you disassociate that primary function from love. be careful of choosing a soulmate. If you have the same purpose and the same devotion to something greater as well as each other, then sure, but understand love is versatile and everywhere. Learn to love yourself, for no one will love you like you, no one will care for you like you. We are alone, regardless of everybody else, we are our own.

Psychology is a science that studies the reaction of matter in complex patterns, in other words, the mind. Reactions of the mind and body via situation and society is the study of psychology which is a legit science. What is most important is not to shun the science, but to ask for the how, and then we with logic can create sustainable patterns of how we truly work and why we work that way.

Superstitions are just that, they are not real, only fueled by coincidence. Mana is simply water, and stamina is simply food. Remember to utilize the self, we are not made to be perpetual we require food; however, we can minimize the amount we need to continue. Some styles will require that you do not give up on eating, and others play well with vegan-based diets or fasting. How you choose to live may determine your style. Also remember that you are carving the body, making it work a specific way, so choose wisely.

Remember that the past is inevitable, what is done is done, the present is where your experience is, and the future is unfathomable until fathomed. If you read this far in this book, your future is unfathomable. Get ready to see it.

It is understood the amount of information given here, so the best way to remember is to create mantras or use mantras on what you need to work on. This can work morally or scientifically. There are many mantras, and much information that could be given, however, the purpose of this book is to be precise. Always further your research on your own. Information that pertains to your path is always the best, don't be afraid to use your resources.

Knowledge

This knowledge will be used throughout the rest of the book. This knowledge is a holder of scientific information, in other words, an easy way to remember lots of information.

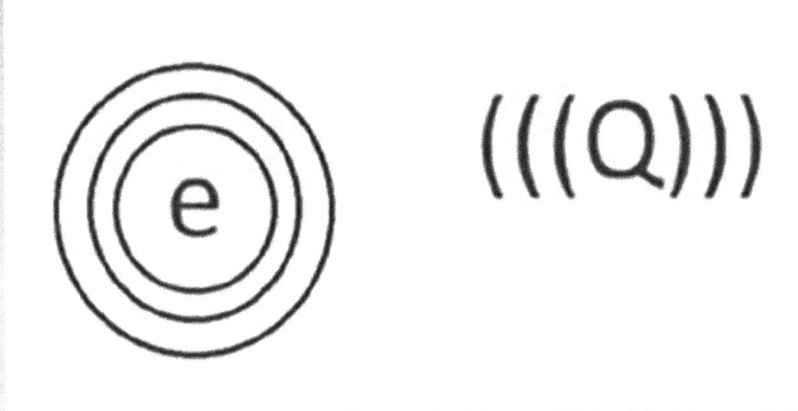

(((E))) was used in ancient times to describe spatial understanding, where the (((Q))) holds the same properties used in modern times to hold an entity within itself (used in possibly real ghosts' videos to keep an entity within the video). To remember spatial understanding, we will use the (((E))). The eh sound represents the self, the internal part of us. The second layer represents our external self and can be represented as ah. The third layer represents our location, or the location of E on a grander scale, represented by the oh sound. The last layer is the representation of what is outside of us within the location, making the u sound. This is another way to see it.

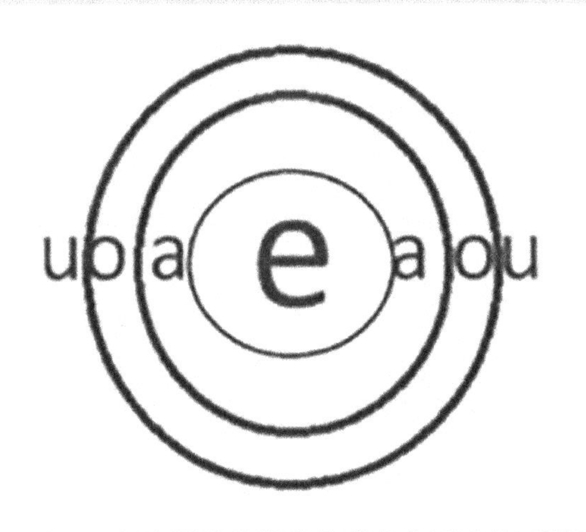

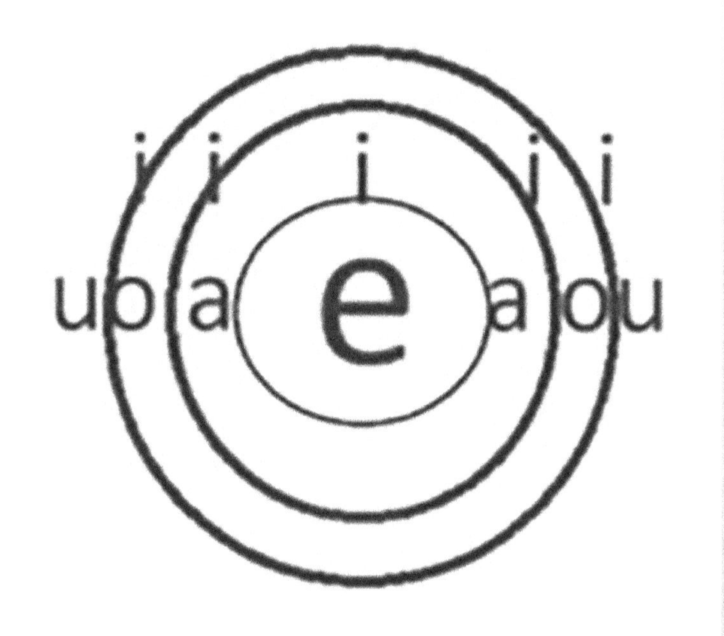

The parenthesis could be represented in which I represent the boundary.

This can be used to represent the self-relativity of an individual. It can further be used to represent barriers of electromagnetic fields. We produce a field of energy with the blood moving through our bodies, as well as the earth, the sun, and the galaxy. The boundaries of space to what we know is at the largest scale a galaxy. This is the literal scale; the galaxies are individuals in space in this representation as the largest. So, the circle of self could be represented as this as well.

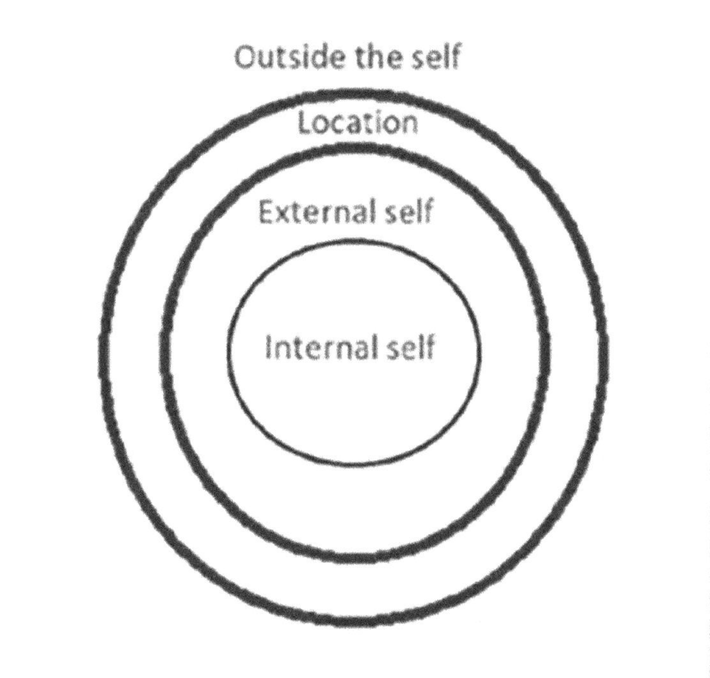

This represents the layers of the circle of self, the following represents the circle of location:

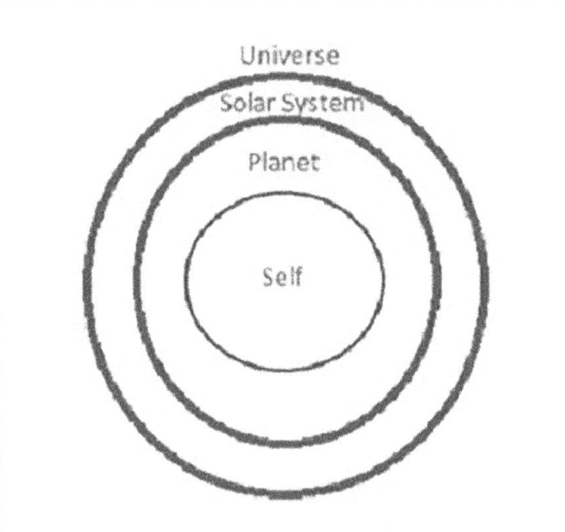

We can fold the circle of self into the circle of location, and layer planet, solar system, and universe to have all self-properties, meaning each can have their own relativity. This is the map of relativity. To remember all of this all you need is this (((E))).

The next section is based on the number system 0-9. This section shows the significance of numbers that give wisdom on their connection that is throughout science and reality.

Zero is significant for nothing, and the most literal nothing is space. There are no negative numbers, they are considered imaginary because they do not exist. While a negative one cannot be drawn geometrically, zero can be. Even though it is nothing it has properties in geometry. The circle has no points, making it zero, however, the constant of a circle is Pi, and Pi is infinite. So, a constant of nothing is infinite. Space, although nothing, is infinite. At least that is one possibility of how space forms itself.

One however, is everything that is not nothing, it is the whole as one. Time runs as a whole, regardless of distance, there is the now, the one whole. There is only one existence. If it is nonexistence, then it is nothing.

Two are the variables of nothing and everything else. The Center of the atomic structure of atoms (other than hydrogen) is the first two electrons. Two allows the extremes of yin and yang, or the hard and the soft, like the rotation of blood through the heart (hard) and the liver (soft). Two allows a rotation. There are also the two things that earth creates, magnetism and gravity, both generated by one, but giving off two properties.

Three is special in how all protons and neutrons are made of three quarks. The quarks are organized in a 2/3 1/3 pattern. From the brain to mathematical equations, electricity, and chemistry we see these patterns.

Four is harder to find. In most cases, 4 things together are a family. One example is the structure of our DNA created by 4 specific chemicals, adenine (A), cytosine (C), guanine (G), and thymine (T).

Five is abstract and harder to see. In a 2/3 1/3 pattern, you have 2 types and 3 parts, making 5. The brain has two hemispheres and the nervous center. The hand has 5, possibly representing the abstraction of our minds, as abstract as that is.

Six is seen in light. There are 6 colors, with clear differentials and borders.

Seven is specialized, simply just a mix of 3 and 4. For example, four chemicals make up DNA and 3 telomeres are holding a strand of DNA together, two ends and one middle.

Eight is a rotation and is seen in the organization. One of the most famous 8 is buddha's divine truths. The 8 has worked on elements the same way the divine truths move. They are separated into two families, two squares to create the 8.

Nine is zooming in and out in three steps each. These sizes up dimensions, from the molecular to the gigantic. However, it is also used in the triforce, when specific variables are used. This triforce holds five equations, using three equilateral triangles, with a total of nine sides, each equation is a problem in electricity.

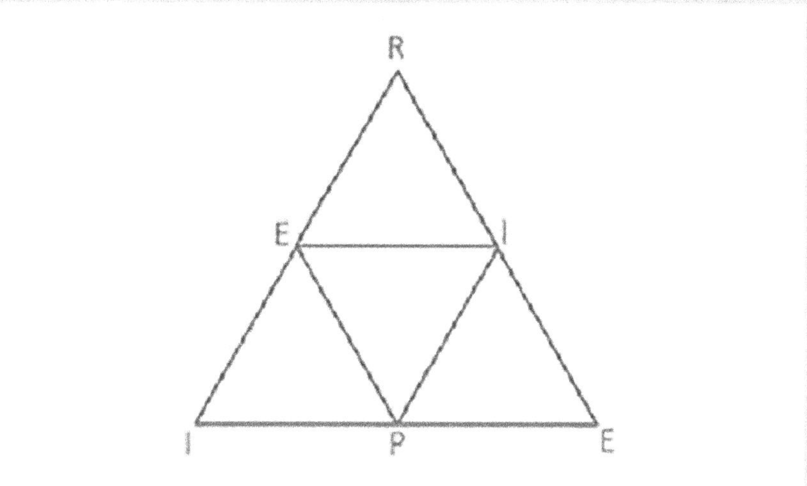

There are five equations, each triangle being one. The three right side up, the one upside down and the edges of the whole create five equations. This is a way to hold this information.

There are various ways to hold information. The best way is through geometry. The first is the 6 made with two triangles. Each triangle holds three movements within the matter that can be manipulated with matter to create results. This is for later on.

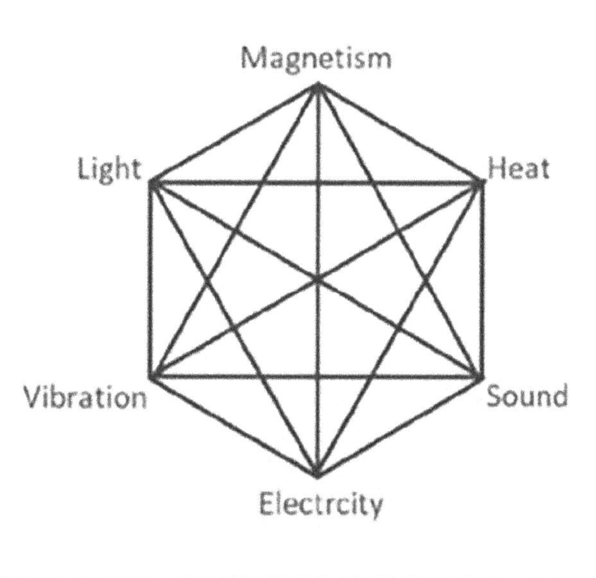

This is a scientific holder, however not as intertwined and convincing as the rest, it is based on molecular movements and equal parts.

Next is the 8, separated into two families. The first family is as follows:

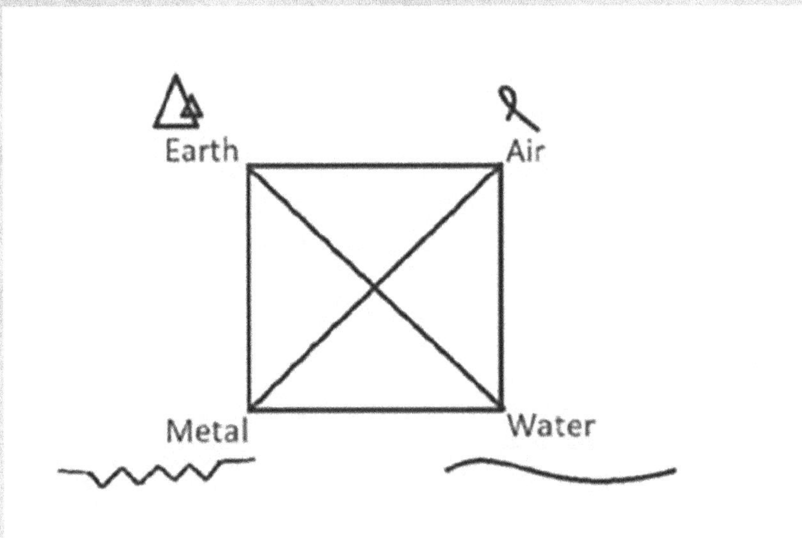

This is the family of states. Earth is represented by a triangle, showing both the molecular to the gigantic shapes of matter. This is the state in which matter is stacked and piled. Air is tumbling within its contained environment representing gaseous states. Water fills and flows representing plasma states and liquid states. Metal can be shaped to a point, or rigid-like, representing the difference between metals and earth.

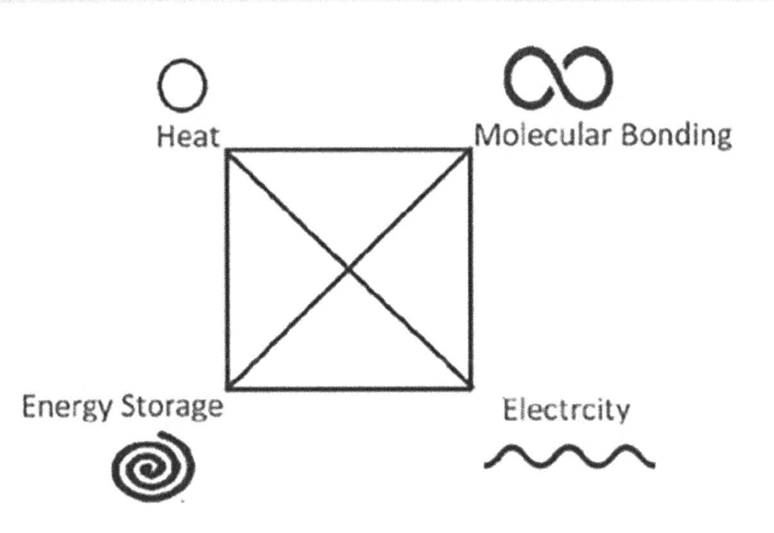

This square is the family of movement. First, we have heat represented by a circle, which represents the outer electron surveillance orbit movement. This represents heat. Molecular bonding is represented by the infinite, which is the bonding process of atoms. Electricity is represented by the circular movement of flow through electron surveillance orbits. The spiral represents the layers of the atom creating a circle movement within, this is energy storage. The final result is as shown:

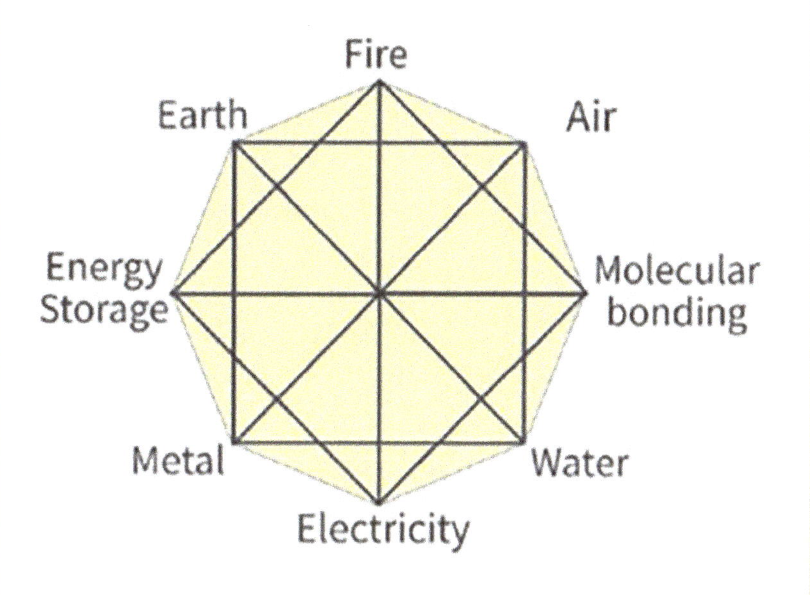

When you make a line between air and metal, it separates the rotation from self-movements to joint movements. When you make a line between water and earth, it separates the rotation from the electrical process and the heat process. When you draw a line from heat to electricity, it separates heat usage to conduction of earth and metal, and the convection of air and water. Also, it separates electricity based on grounding types and conductive types. When you draw a line from energy storage to molecular bonding, it separates the transmutation process of metal and the process of earth forming. This process is seen further in values of 2, like light and dark, so nothing something, 0 and 1.

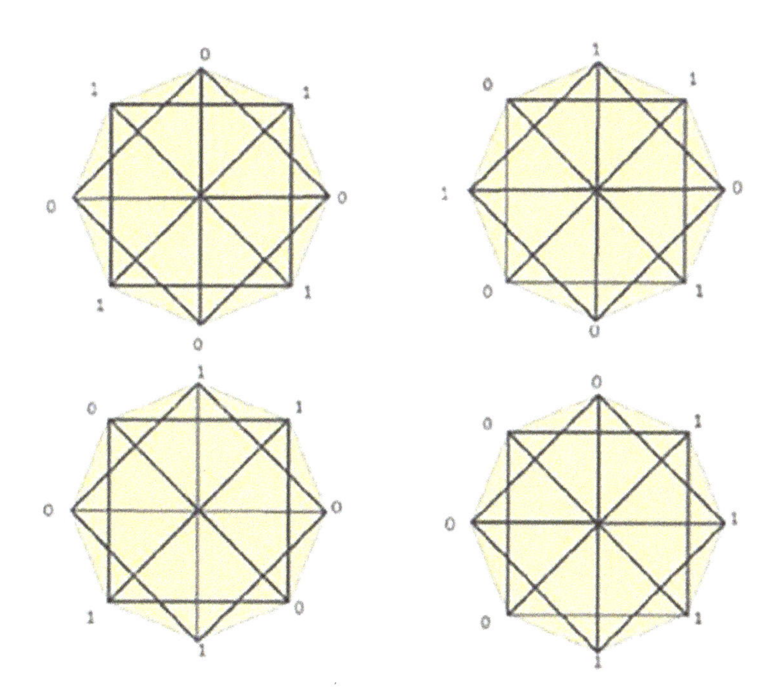

When cut in half the first circle represents the same and the opposite when cutting in either direction. The others cut either the same or the opposite. These octagonal matrices have only so many patterns, these being the four patterns.

Chemical 8 is based on a 01101001 pattern. When you make an 8-pointed star, we get a chemical process. The movement family is either a give or a-take movement, where the matter family each has a give and a take.

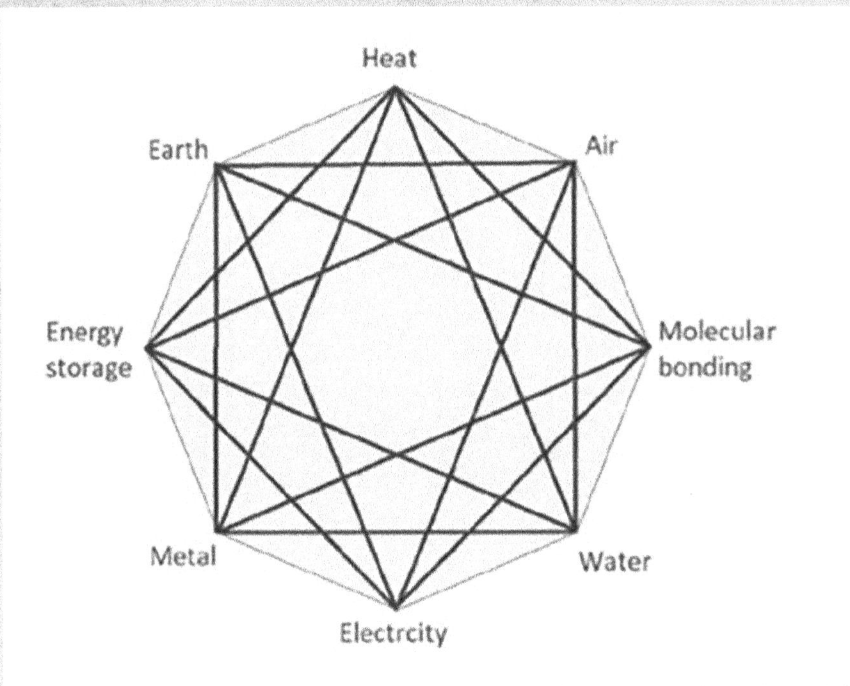

The family of movement is the key. Electricity grounds to earth and air, attracted to or giving to those two, whereas heat gives to metal and water. The two most natural expressions of light within our atmosphere are fire and lighting, The two together give and create light. Energy storage requires water and air to be achieved, like in batteries or with our bodies.

Blood is required to pump, and breathing is required as well during sleep, granting a charge. Molecular bonding requires earth and metal. Think of this like eating and digestion. This is the darkness, the eternal movements, like the color black, the absorption of. Earth has both gives and takes the same with air metal, and water. This is the chemical star.

The chemical star also gives a representation of the chakras in a new system. Each point is a full body layer to the center. This layer system is not the same as the chakra system. The chakra system can be represented as the final layer, the endocrine system. The top layers are as follows, from the bottom up, and outside in.

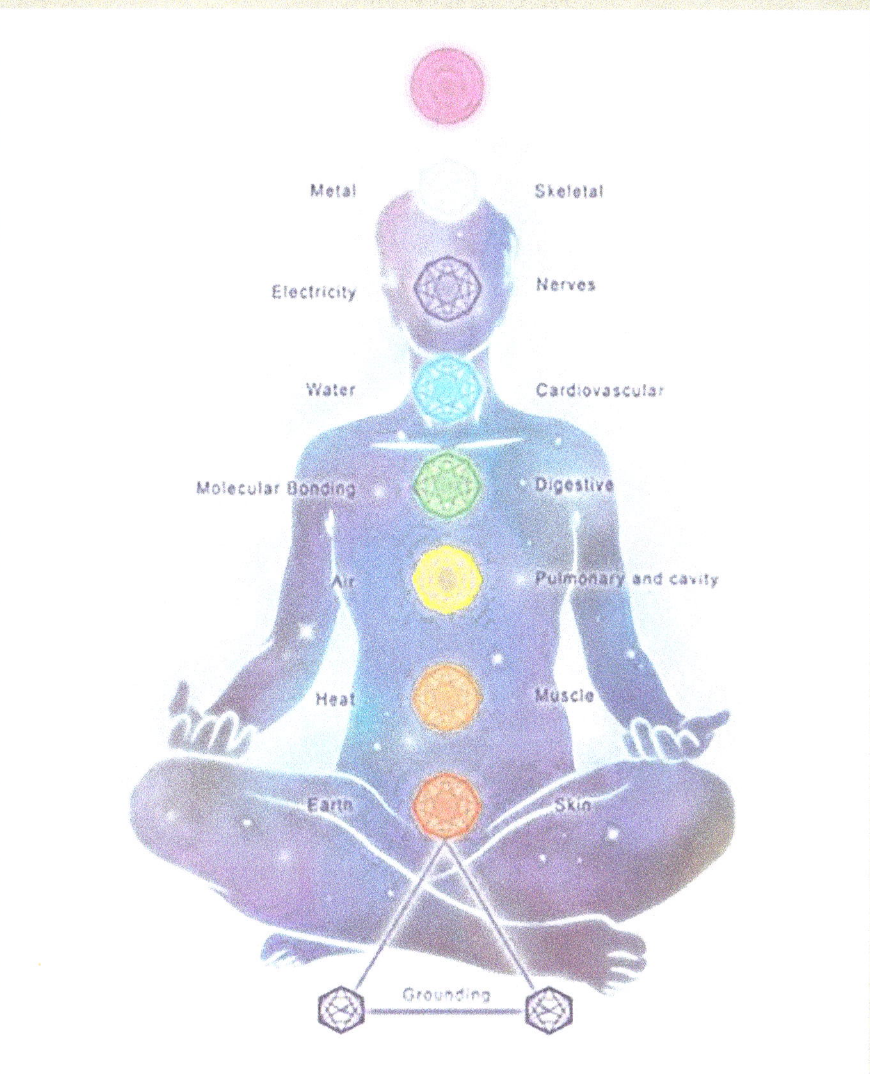

Earth represents the skin, based on its heat absorption, and most earth tends to have a reddish hew. Fire tends to have an orange color, and muscle has properties of burning energy, this is the next layer, muscle. Air in a light bulb gives off a yellow color and represents the next layer, the chest and stomach cavities, and the pulmonary system. Green tends to be seen in plant life and represents the recycling of energy in the digestive system that is within the cavity. The blue represents water and the cardiovascular system, which feeds the rest of the body with the digestive system. Purple represents electricity and the nervous system, which regulates the heart and all other systems. The deepest layer is the skeletal system, represented as metal. The next system is the charge and the endocrine system which goes back down and back up on the chakras that we know of.

Each chakra point is a pool point of energy created by related endocrine-connected chemical dispensers more or less. Now we have simultaneous layers working together, however, we can go further in by adding more rotations. Each point of the second rotation is in between two points. They represent a process that makes two more families. These are the first four families.

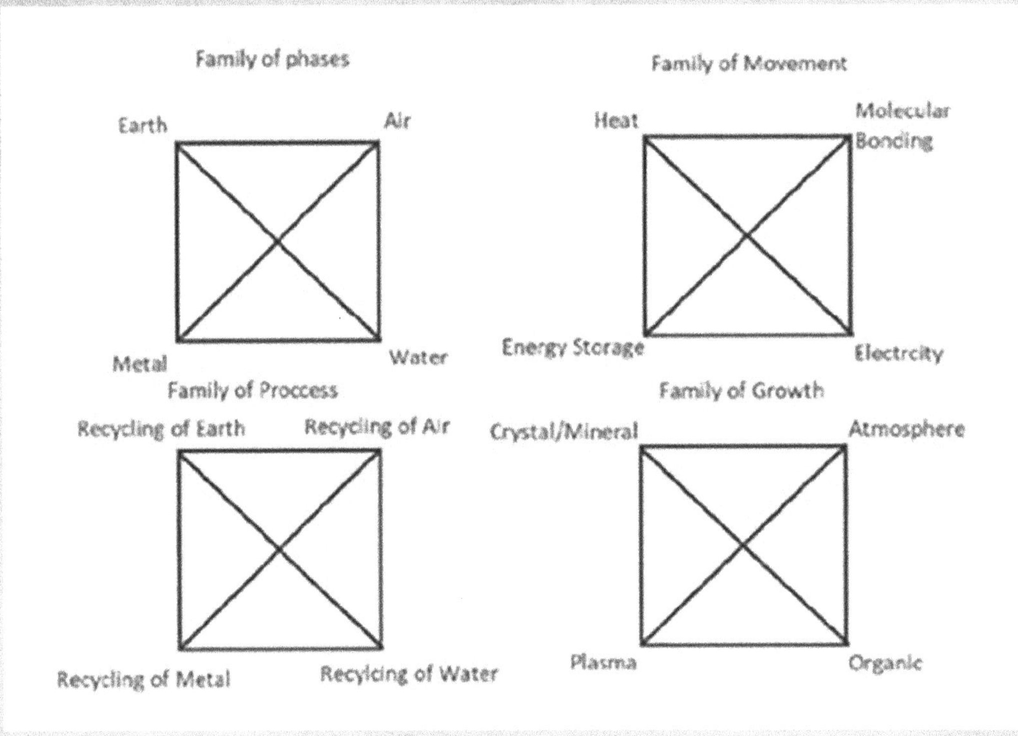

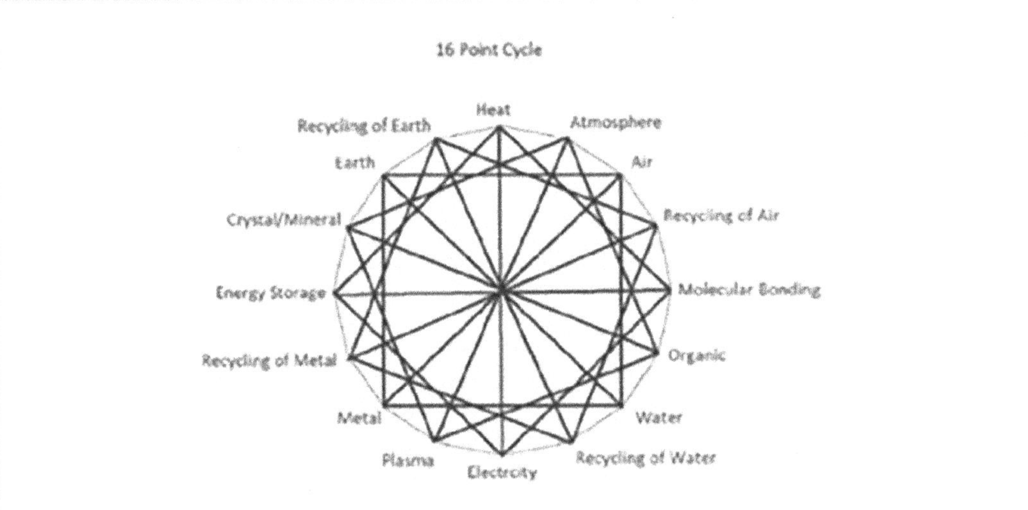

The family of processes and the family of growth both are the combination of the first rotation. If you go further, you get more of the process in which the elements react, using the rotation of creation, made by the family of growth, and the rotation of deconstruction, made by the family of processes, which further gives to the spiral in which the order moves from earth to energy storage, meaning this process has a specific direction in which it moves.

The family of processes adds the 4 inner systems. Recycling of earth represents eating and digesting, recycling of water represents drinking and urinating, recycling of air represents breathing in and out, and recycling of metal represents sleeping and awake.

The family of growth represents the outer senses. Crystal and minerals represent touch and feel, the atmosphere represents hearing and balance, organic represents smell and taste, and plasma represents sight and depth. Here we see these systems in a full anatomy based circle.

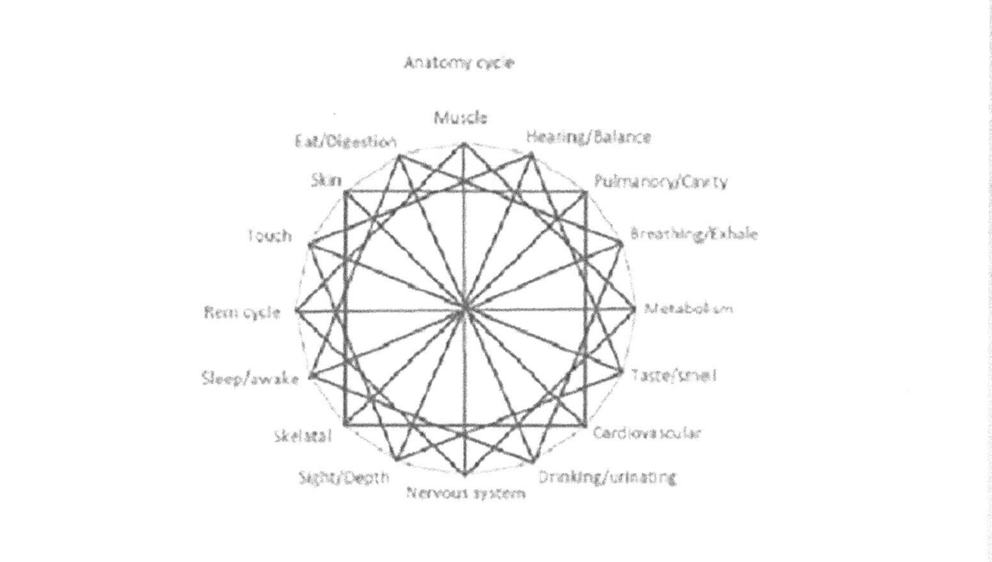

These rotations can also retain in other systems. If you take the Family of processes and follow their square, each line would represent a process of science. Recycling of earth to recycling of air gives the process of meteorology (the science of weather). Recycling air to Recycling water gives a process of biology (the science of life). The recycling of water to the recycling of metal is a process of metallurgy (the science of metals). Recycling of metal to recycling of earth is a process of geology (earth science).

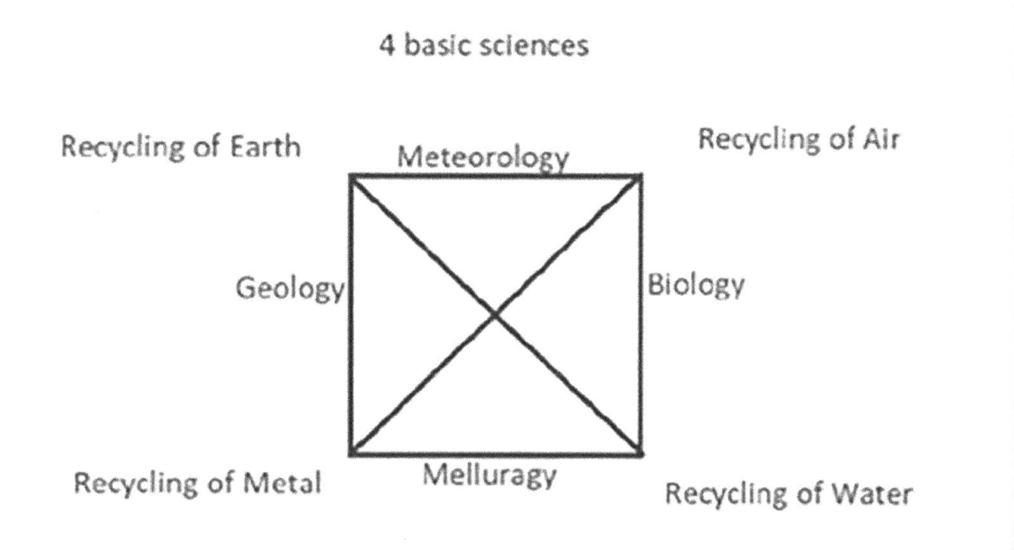

This is all new and yet lines up with natural science. They hold information, so these families are learning the steps of how information is held. There are many more representational families that can cause rotations. Some examples are feelings, the process Crystal information, further movements, and so on. These other squares are in deeper studies. The basics are all that are needed for now. However, the significance of the family of 18 is also a way to remember energy.

The values of 666, 288, 963, 576, and 864 are all 18. The significance of these sets is how they relate to energy. 666 is represented by a darker shade of the primary colors, the primary shade, and a lighter shade of the primary colors. 288 represents the first three lines of the periodic table of elements. 963 was significant in Tesla's research and represents the relation of electromagnetism. 576 represents the 7 keys, 5 sharps, and 12 together value of 6, representing sound. 864 is significant for its representation of the acute, equilateral, and obtuse triangles, in relation to there stars. 369 is in the structure of energy created in microbiology, the life force energy created in the mitochondria.

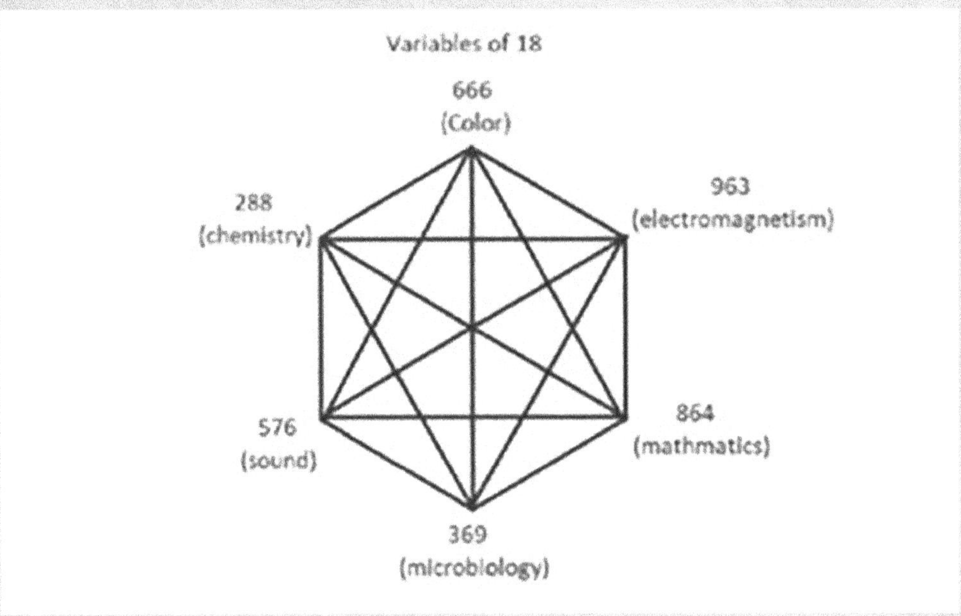

Each value represents light, electromagnetism, sound, geometry, microbiology, and chemistry. These are abstract connections, however, used in further study.

The significance of nine is in the Norse, Chinese and Celtic seeds of life. The Celtic and Norse are related, and the Chinese its own. When researching info, they seem to come in threes, two similar and one different but the same, a 2/3 1/3 pattern that can be used to analyze data.

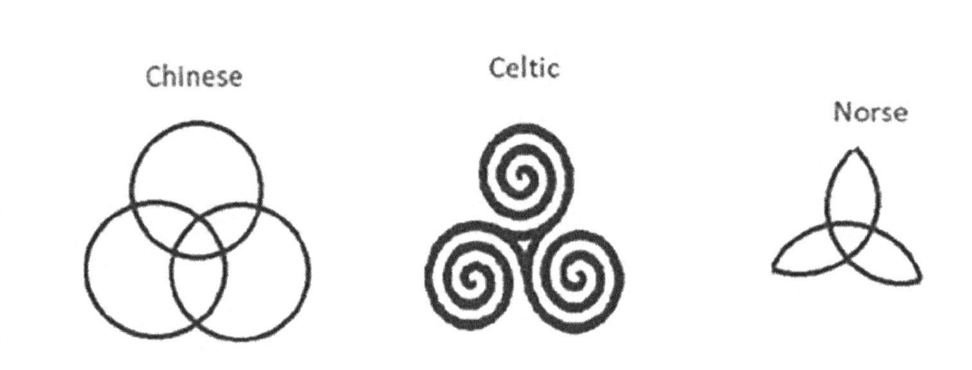

The best use of this system is in the triforce-based pattern with 5 triangles that were referenced earlier. The following can be used to hold information about space.

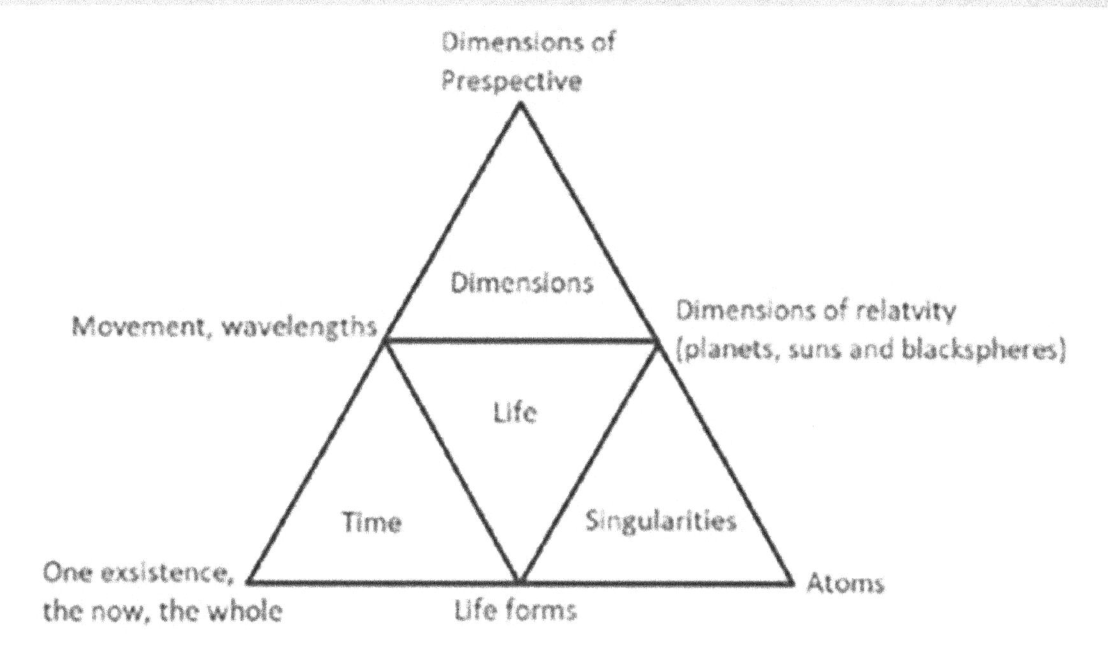

Each triangle has three ways to calculate the primary triangle. Each point used to connect to another triangle has two points that are similar to each other making it a 2/3 point. Each endpoint is considered a one-third point.

The triangle of time has three values of the time. One way to calculate time is movement and distance. The second way is that all are at the same time, however, separated by the first variable in distance and movement. The third is that the only thing that cares about time, is organic life.

The triangle of relativity is simply that which makes a field around itself or within itself. Organic life has the heart beating, creating a field, atoms naturally have electron barriers, and planets or stars create magnetic fields to sustain life when they are big enough.

The triangle of dimensions is based on perspective, in other words, the mind, or point of view. but literal dimensions are created by celestial and planetary gravity, and by wavelengths created by movement.

The triangle of life is created by movement, planetary relativity, and life itself to further create more life. These are the conditions to create life, however, held together by the last triangle.

The fifth triangle is the perspective of the universe from a molecular standpoint to an astronomical standpoint. These all together create the Triforce. It is good to remember these triangles, it is a good way to hold information.

Another version of holding information together is using the 8 and scientific law, based on the 8 elements.

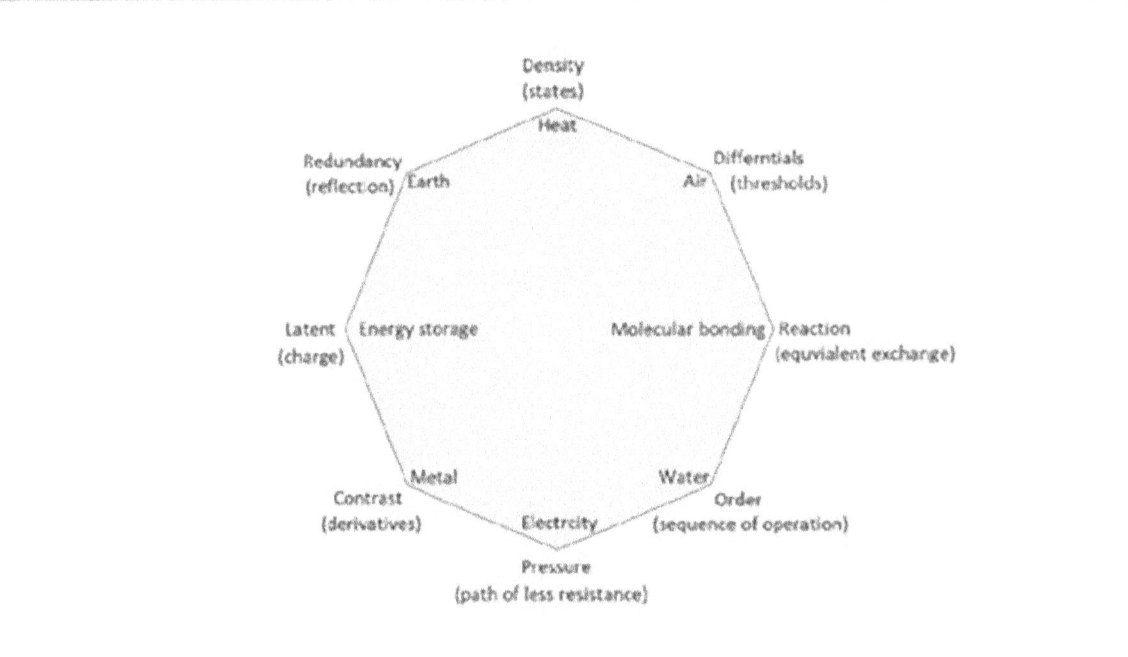

Each law is represented by an aspect of an element. Remember there are many rotations, so this is used to remember the law. Yours may look different, however, remember each law is represented by elemental representation. This is more of an abstract law holder; however, the first law holder is always the elements themselves.

The last symbol that holds knowledge is a little more abstract and holds knowledge within its pattern.

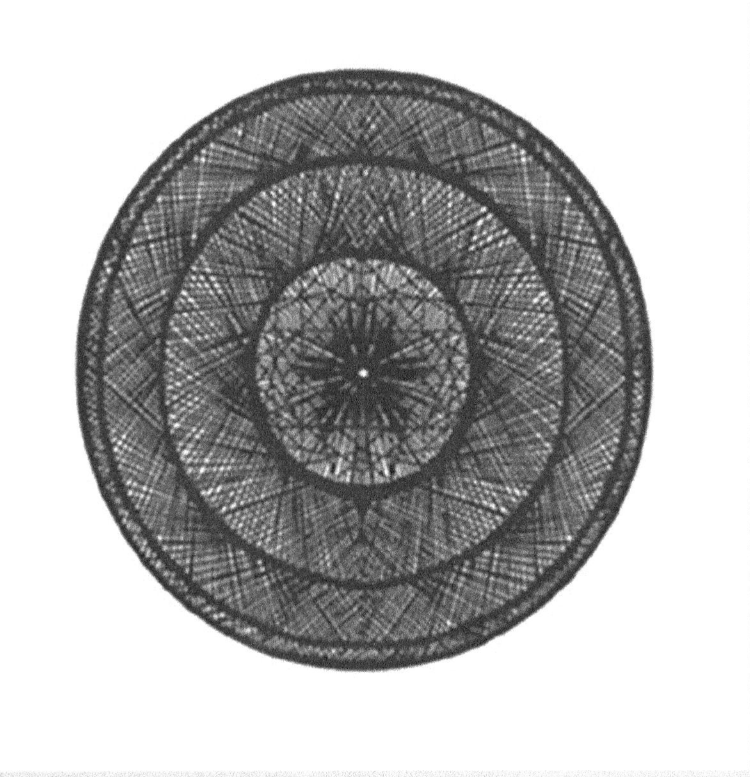

This is a 192-pointed star. This star is significant because of the multiples within it. There are only so many numbers with high multiples. This number contains numbers associated with the periodic table. Other numbers that go with the periodic table are 288 and 576. You can look at the multiples to understand further how they are associated.

The significance of this pattern is the geometrical alignment which allows an actual view of the electron surveillance orbit of copper and silver. It naturally creates a threshold within the number, allowing us to also see the setup of a planet's core. The illusion that is given off by the star is both an inward spiral and a sphere, like a core. At a specific level, we have both gravity and magnetism which move like a spiral and a sphere. It is used as a mental focus and clears illusions. This star will be used further in the book.

Tuning in to you

The best way to understand or hold this information is to do it from your perspective. below are two triangles, each one is a specific pattern, normal, and inverted. Look at all both with a different perspective (flip the book if needed) to find the triangle that best suits you.

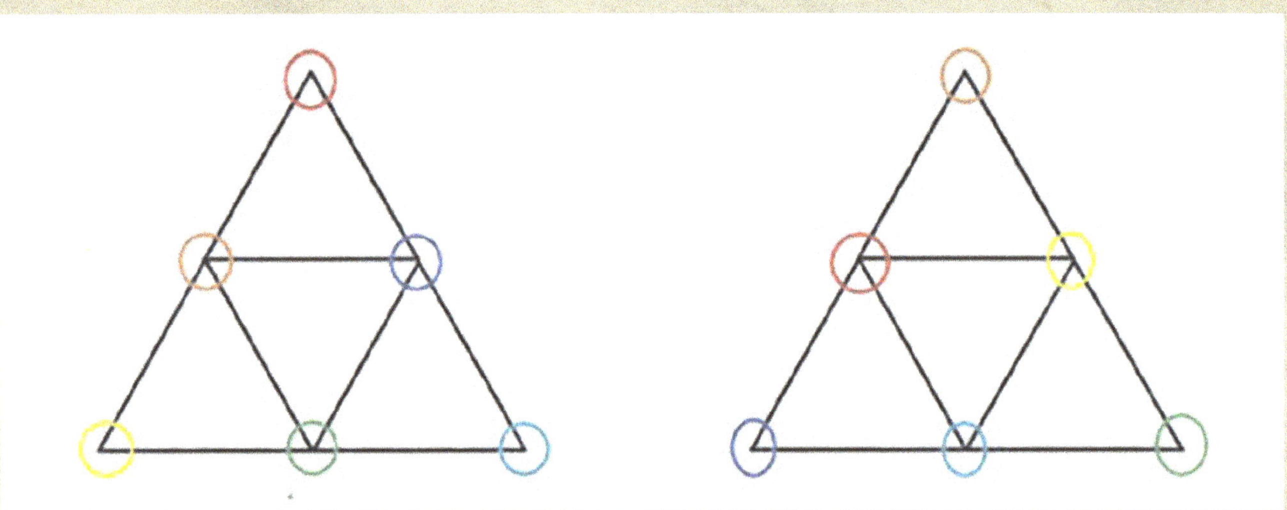

Color can tell a lot about a person, so choose the one that seems like you or the pattern that you are drawn to the most, with the color you prefer up top. Now if you look at the triangles not as a point but as a flat side that you like the most, that is normal for specific types of minds. These patterns are natural and have elemental as well as color meanings.

There are so many meanings for color, what is given now is just a few meanings of the order and the color and what it may tell about you.

Red represents the reality base of an individual, orange represents passion, and yellow can represent pride and curiosity, while green represents kindness, blue represents honesty, and purple represents peace. Each color has an excess of or a lack of one represented as white and the other dark. In other words, each color has a downside and an upside, the goal is to be balanced in each color, meaning your chakras form both light and dark in each color as a Ying and yang.

Next, we have another mind-understanding tool. Using the alchemical star, we will see your personality types. There are 16 combos, each giving a perspective of your being. In this one, rather than what you like, you are going to choose what makes the most sense to you. Which pattern direction makes it easy to understand? We have a normal and flipped version. Take the book and move the book until you have the element on top of which makes the most sense to you. The elements rotate with your body, meaning the top part is your mind, and the rotation to the left is your heart element. This gives two possible choices allowing you to understand that in one direction the relationship between mind and heart is an amplifier, and in the other a recycler. Amplifiers have for example an air heart and a heat mind, meaning their emotions govern their mind, where as an earth heart and heat mind's emotions are governed by the mind not the heart. Choosing a mind is like finding the self, but figuring out the heart is establishing that connection. So, the left octagon would represent the rotation for a natural recycler, and the right one would represent a natural amplifier.

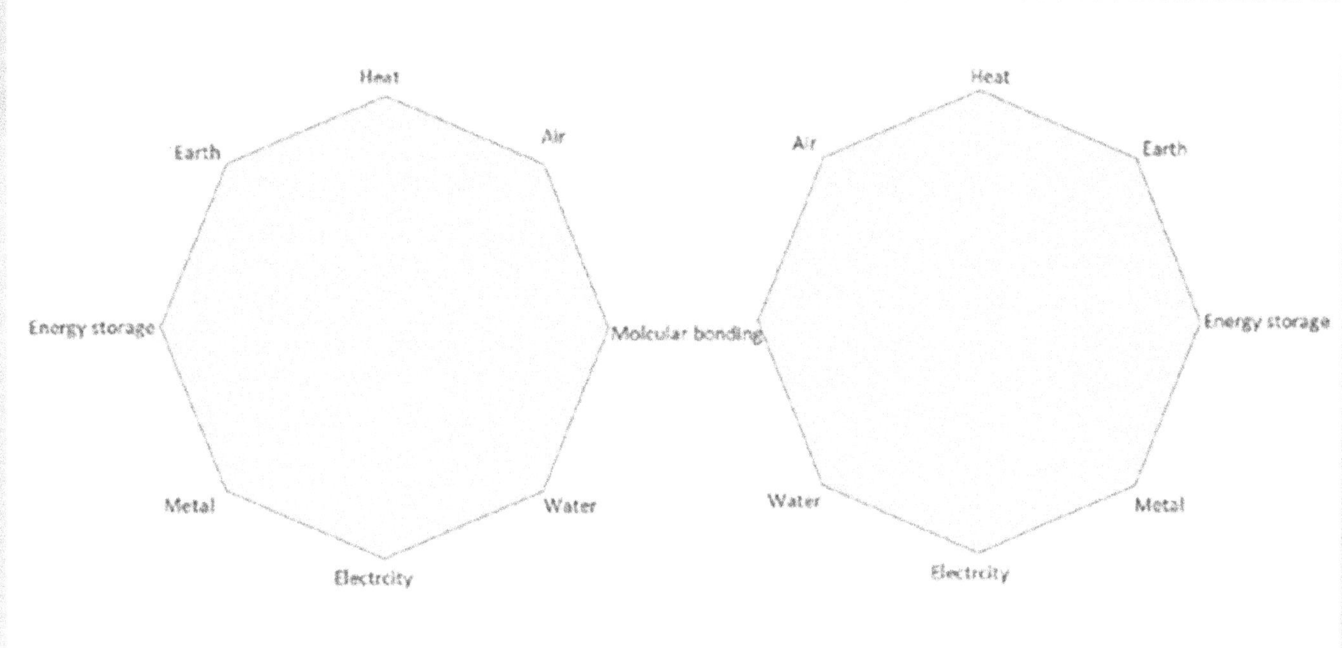

Basics

Here is some information before we begin. You have full access to your brain. When you unlock the brain, you will not gain super calculations, you will not become smarter. In order to grasp the full unlocking of the brain you must understand that the brain is mostly based of action, sensory, and order. Learning the order of things or understanding patterns requires repetition of information. The information given above will allow access to information readily, this will naturally increase you processing power. This will also help with diagnostics, and understanding things by organizing your information, and when you organize you naturally create space for more memory. The next step in unlocking the brain is understanding combo sensory. Your sensory is all interconnected. You can feel something while smelling or seeing already, so to understand combo sensory is to understand the intersection of sensory in the brain already. Meaning if it wasn't possible there would be no place for the extra sensory in the brain, but there is. Therefore, extra sensory is possible. Understand that these extra senses are simply combinations of the senses you already have. Unlocking the brain takes time, however, is not impossible. Remember, the difference between you, geniuses, billionaires, and even gods are simply information you don't have. For example, answers to higher IQ problems are usually just information that you have never been exposed to. Understanding this will allow you to further yourself as an individual. These following techniques will give you a basis to opening the mind, and to further explore the realm of magic.

Read through every one of the basic techniques before practicing. After reading, follow the technique instructions. Please practice your basics before choosing a style.

Meditation Process

This process is key in basic training. This skill is the first step into going further in the mystic arts. Mastery of this skill takes time, however, with a paved road, the time is reduced significantly. What took years of others' mastery, can take weeks to days for a new student to learn how to master. Always be patient, in retrospect, this takes a small portion of your time, and in the end, when done right becomes very enjoyable.

Meditation-

Read through these basics before attempting. Each session should be at least a day apart. Try to make meditation part of your life, once a day for 30 mins, before bed. Not every session should be for a response.

The basics of meditation are in the breath. Sit in an upright position, hands on the knees, and breath in through the nose, while breathing in through the nose feel all that afflicts you, breath out through the top of the mouth, and feel the release through the pallet of your mouth. You can do this to get rid of anxiety, anger, or even just tension in the body. Do this while meditating, in the nose out the mouth. Feel the release and continue breathing like this through the process.

Next focus on your feet, and feel your toes relax, then your feet, ankles, all the way up to your head. Feel the relaxation, remember this feeling. While you breath in feel your toes, and on exhale feel them relax, all the way to the head. Once you do this the first time you should be able to do this faster in other sessions. Now, after you relax every part of your body feel your whole body relax together. Once you have relaxed, focus your attention on just your breathing again.

Do the following the first time you meditate:

3a. While you are breathing, focus simultaneously on your inner eyelids. Now focus on this for the rest of the meditation. You will start to fall asleep and hold your position while nodding off. The result should be a fluctuation of color in the inner eyelids, which is the movement of the inner mind. This color and movement represent you. You have seen your soul. The colors represented are like the elements. Once you know your inner elements you now know how to focus. This may take up to 30 mins. If you lose focus start from step one again.

The following is done for the next step of meditation.

2b. Prayer is used in meditation; however, meditation is used for receiving an answer. Pray is used for creating a direction. First pray with emotion on something like to be worthy of a greater answer, for redemption. You can also pray to feel love again, to gain direction in life, or to find purpose. The answer is always within. After you feel the emotion take over you are ready for an answer. Use step one to get to a meditative state. Fall into sleep once you have established a meditative state.

The following is done for advanced meditation:

3b. Once you are in a relaxed state when you start to nod off, wake yourself back to the meditation state, then go back into sleep and wake yourself again, and gain a balance of both the dream and conscious state at the same time. This is the median. To go further access yourself by asking something like your greatest fear, see your greatest fear, then allow the dream to reveal you're true greatest fear. It will scare you, but release the fear while staying in a meditative state, it cannot harm you unless it is there, you are alone, and fear is in the moment, let go of fear. Now fall into sleep. This is the step to opening the chakra points. When it first occurs, you will feel like you have streams of energy leaving the body. it will feel like an antenna, use the connection, by wiggling your neck to cross the streams above you. They will connect and create an orb; this orb will give you the connection to the greater universe. It is an abstract connection, and one can receive it once this is established. This is the higher connection.

Before you meditate more after this point, you should advance the self-further.

Another way to advance meditation is through dreaming. Once you establish a medium balance, you should have more control over sleeping and dreaming. When existing in a dream you can hold your state in the medium and even change your dream and go back to sleep.

Biofield Manipulation

We create a natural field of wavelengths around us. There are aggressive ways to manipulate the biofield and passive aggressive. This will cover two passive-aggressive ways to affect your biofield.

Kaioken-

This is a body technique. First, relax your bicep, and feel your body's relaxation, if you have not done meditative relaxation, you may not know the sensation. Relax the bicep, then flex the bicep, while flexing, relax the bicep, this should allow the blood to fill your muscles further. Then release and feel your muscle go back to size. It may feel sore when you allow this to happen this is normal. You can do this in any part of your body.

Another way to use this technique is to do this while using weights. Watch out not to pull or tear anything, start with lower weights when using the technique. The power comes with time and doing this often gives great results.

Cross streaming-

This is a body technique. First, get in a horse stance. Tighten body, and strike, crossing the body during the strike, while lifting the opposite leg at the same time. Do this with the other side and repeat back and forth between sides. Do this as fast as you want, you must keep tense. After about ten times, pull into a standing position, hands over one another, and release tension. Move hands in ball form around each other, while moving them in and out from each other. You should feel the magnetism of your biofield.

Another way to do this is to wave the arms around and make sure you cross in front and back to cross-stream your energy. Then touch your fingers to each other, and then move them apart and you should get the same result. This does not require tension and is a quick way to raise some ki.

Third Eye Evolution

The physical third eye is an observatory tool. Using the third eye allows us to see the movements of our biofields, like seeing auras, and further seeing our stories. The best use of the third eye is paired with our feeling, to allow us to see the flow of energy in another. These are the basic steps to opening and evolving the self, with the use of the third eye.

Third eye strengthening-

This is a mind-body technique. Have another person stand in front of a white wall. Stare at a person's forehead for about 10 seconds without blinking, then look at the person's nose. Within your peripheral you should see a hue around the person, this is their aura, the color can tell many things about what is being used in the person, or what they are expressing. This technique takes practice and varies from person to person.

Another technique is to hold your hand in front of you in between some light. Hold your hand to the light, and blink 5 times fast, hold close on 5th blink. You should get a hue of your hand and should see your hand outline by the light. This is practicing seeing residue light. Use this technique to focus on your aura-seeing abilities.

Third eye awakening-

This is a mental technique. Use a cross-stream form before doing this. Take a charged hand and put it 6 inches from the nose. Make small circles while moving your hand up towards your forehead, no closer than one inch. Close your eyes and let your body feel the circle of your hand near your head, then press your hand against your forehead and rub your hand in small circles on your forehead. This should unlock the third eye. Now do some Third eye strengthening.

The result may vary, but for the most part, you are opening your inner mind, which should allow you to see further than color. There are some rules to using this. What you see is a description of the being, use truth and you will see the truth. Understanding the truth is not what we determine, it moves with imagination, and cannot be fathomed, therefore we use imagination with truth to see. Do not determine anything, it is already determined what it is.

If you wish to explore this further, understand the representation of elements to read. Also understand that it may mean familiarity, similarity, the era of, it, the rumor of, student of, purpose, or witness to. Remember to feel your way through, understand what you are, and a place to come back to. Remember you are reading a journey, what is done is done, and what can be done has not occurred yet. Further on reading later.

Always give time before using another mind technique.

Mindscape Building

These techniques allow the exploration of your inner mind and turn it into a valuable tool. Sometimes enhancing the mind can be an extreme change, it is good to do these techniques with time in between each technique. These are advanced techniques, those that are ready will understand the use of the mind's eye technique on their own. Each situation is different; however, the use of the mind's eye is to see around you with greater senses.

Mind's eye technique-

This is a mental technique. This unlocks full body sensory. Look at the space behind you, then close your eyes and see the space in your inner mind. You are seeing the space in which is behind you and seeing it within your mind. Now feel the space behind you. You should be able to tell if people are moving. Feel the vibration in the air, or the premunition of movement, that can be calculated. Allow what is there to move you when it moves. You can do this by having someone behind you choose a hand to move, then sense which hand is being used. Trust your instinct and do this without want, do this with a neutral feeling. Try this in various spaces. You may have to reset by seeing the space and seeing it within your inner mind.

Charged meditation-

This is a mental technique. This is not a shortcut, best to do this after several successful meditations. This is a three-day process.

First, use cross-streaming to charge yourself. Close your eyes while doing this. Put your hand 3 inches above your head and start to do circles. Rotate your hand down to the base of the skull, still not touching the head. Take both hands, placed on either side of your head, by your ears, still 3 inches away. Circle till you get to the base of the skull. Now use one hand 3 inches away from the back of the head. Circle and get closer to the head, till the hand is touching. Then rub the spot till you feel a pain in the back of the head or lightheadedness. If you do it right, you should feel pain in your head, and it will last for about three days.

Your meditation should become charged, and relaxing, this will allow you to do shallow meditation and access the medium easier.

The mind negative-

This is a mental technique. Understanding our metaphysical physiology is understanding the true routes of our energy and understanding how they are sustained. We are always at around 98 degrees Fahrenheit; we are born able to sustain this temperature. Our bodies create memory partly due to the molecular structure being heated. The longer we live over time the more powerful our memories become.

The mind negative is the place where you imagine in your head. This space is created by the heat negative of the body in the brain, much like taking a picture. Sight is another extreme that allows for helping feed memory. This is the eternal negative, and the heat must be there for the receptors to do their job to create the negative.

Imagining outside of the self requires a reflection of the image within on the outside of you, meaning even your point of view or location. This is how it can be described:)(((E)))(, the outside of the self, a reflection on the outside of your consciousness. Reflecting on the mind's negative is simply like making your imagination around you, which can be done at a young age for some. Just imagine a character, like a ninja, jumping from sign to sign or tree to tree. This is exercising the mind's negative.

Boundary Understanding

These techniques vary in usage; however, all have to do with strengthening your connection to sound. These are vital techniques for several sorcery styles. You should try all techniques, and in the end, evaluate which is strongest for you. Usually, that is the style you can use the best.

Inner voice tuning-

This is an inner mind technique. Place your hands over your mouth in a cup formation. Speak into it and hear your voice echo. Close your eyes and think some words, now say the words in your hands, hear the echo, and make your inner voice echo those words. This is a difficult technique and may require hearing louder echoes of your voice.

Next, you can whisper or scream and hear your voice in either direction, loud or quiet. Now use your inner voice and make it louder or quieter.

These techniques are used to clear the mind physically. The next technique is used to put the mind in sync with the body. Sit down and get in a meditative stance. Humm the ah sound. While humming, hum with your inner mind at the same time. This will cause a connection between your mind and voice; it will feel like a click.

This last technique is more advanced but starts using the inner mind more. Think of a sound in your head. Make it as real as possible, like wind blowing, water rushing, fire burning, wood growing, metal scrapping, thunder rumbling, or rocks tumbling. Whatever sound you can make in your head that sounds exactly like the sound in real life is closer to you than anything else. If you don't know the sound, go listen to it. Clearer sounds tend to have these effects in meditation. That sound that is clearest is your tool or weapon to use. It also suggests the element to which you are closest. Get creative with that sound, make that element move in different ways and see if you can hear it clearly in your head. This is the inner mimic technique.

Spatial tuning-

This is a sensory technique. This technique is sound based. Using the vowels in the (((E))), we can understand spatial tuning based on the movement of the sound made by each vowel.

First get into a meditative position, close your eyes, and hum the eh sound. Feel the vibration of the eh. It should feel like an inner vibration within the mouth and lungs. Now hum the ah sound. You'll notice the range of vibration is now off the inner cheek of the mouth. Now hum the oh sound. You will notice the oh sound is more pushed out of the body. Now hum the sound. You will notice slight vibration in the lips with a more intense push.

You can use this technique with the inner mind in sync humming technique to feel another range of vibration with the vowels. Also, try changing from vowel to vowel to exercise your awareness of vibration or the changes in the vibration.

Humming skin technique-

This is a sensory technique. There are three variations to this technique. All can be applied together.

First, when you use the eh sound, feel the vibration of the air in your lungs by making a higher pitched eh sound. The vibration in the air in the body can also travel down to the lungs. Put your hand on your sternum and hum, you should feel the vibration traveling in the lungs as well. This is the first variation.

The second variation is feeling the vibration of the sound on the skin. Use the ah sound to connect with your skin. Feel the vibrations move through the body as if the vibration is flowing through water, your jing or flesh. The other vowels flow through you differently, however, can be used with this technique. U tends to move away from you. Channel the sound by feeling the flow of vibration through your arm and allow it to channel to your palm by relaxing and allowing internal vibrations from the sound to flow through you internally and externally.

The third variation channels through the mind. Play some music on headphones, and here the song plays in your head. There are two ways to do this. First, make the song in your inner mind sound just like the song. Meditate and feel the connection of your inner mind with the rest of your nervous system. You can play the vibration in a specific spot knowing that electrically you are connected to your entire body at once. You can hon in on a spot and feel the vibrations leave your body as the song plays.

The second way to do this is to use the inner ear. This requires listening to the whole of the song at once. Meaning every instrument that is playing at once you are paying attention to. This will connect you to your inner ear when achieved, allowing vibration to flow on the oh sound, meaning you can connect with the area around you. This is an active listening technique.

The third way to use the inner ear is to pull on both earlobes while listening. You can open access to the whole of your ear this way, and while meditating will naturally allow the sound to travel through the body.

Qi Connections

These techniques focus on full-body connections that are already there. Focus causes a redundancy, allowing you to strengthen the technique, when you know what you are focusing on causes a natural redundancy which again strengthens the technique. Here are some qi techniques.

Free flow technique-

This is a body mental technique. Heat rises, and we are at a constant 98 degrees Fahrenheit. We create a flow through our blood vessels that spreads heat throughout our bodies evenly. Our nervous system travels downward grounding within our bones, to stabilize an electromagnetic field. With these systems combined, we have our true metaphysics. Heat goes up, electricity flows down. With eyes closed feel this technique, put your fists out in front of you, now lift them and feel the assertion of your field when you put them down, about halfway with a sudden stop. This is the free flow technique, feeling the multiple simultaneous systems at work.

The all-connect-

This is a relaxation technique. Our bodies are made of mostly water, flesh, and bone essentially. This is called que Jing, which is a word that describes our flesh. Water ripples and so does our movement. We can allow sound and vibration to move throughout the body, not just where we channel it. The body is fully connected, in multiple simultaneous patterns, electrical, mechanical, and chemical all working to react and make the body react. Emotions will affect you on a whole scale, that is why we feel anger in more than one part of the body, same with love, sorrow, and joy. Instinct and listening are very all connected. We can use the mind to give us further connection, and even program ourselves with thought and movement. This works as we mix in the emotions as well.

One example of programming is through martial arts. As you do it more it becomes a whole reaction, which reprograms our fear reaction to instill a reaction to it. by defending against the punch, and gaining arm control, like in jujitsu, we reprogram the body by performing the simplest of tasks over and over until the body remembers the move. You can do this with many martial arts, but also the mystic arts with meditation, channeling, and other techniques.

As we can include detail in a move, like small adjustments to perfect a strike, we can include detail with meditation and other things. The key to any of this in detail, and to understand greater detail is to understand science.

Zen pose-

This is a meditation technique. Get into a meditative pose. Next, close your eyes, and feel your arms. You are trying to make a complete circuit, creating yourself into a load. The feeling can come in many forms, the most natural is a focus. When you find your load pose, you will feel focused, it's like a subtle click. Move your hands around each other, until you feel the clarity of focus. It doesn't matter what hand signs you use; however, the best is usually compensation for the body to create the load.

Usually, a path of less resistance can be shaped by injury and emotion. If you find yourself moving when tuning in, you may want to clear yourself by channeling down the arms. One way to detect the load is to use a crystal quartz pendulum tuned into the actual movement of the body. When you find your Zen pose the pendulum will be completely still. It is easier to find someone else's, however possible to find your own. This will be covered for those that are interested later.

Hidden Techniques

These techniques are used to hide oneself, whether you are hiding your wavelengths or your presence. These are also used to hide while you're working on another so that you can avoid reactions from other people. Hiding presence-

This is a wavelength technique. That means that this focuses on the body's natural wavelengths created by the heart and blood.

To hide your presence, you must use the cross-stream technique first. Next, hold your hands 6 inches away from each other, move to 3 inches apart, move to 5 inches apart, then move to 2 inches apart and fold your hands into the body. Due 6 3 5 2 quickly then turn your hands into the body. This hand movement will balance your wavelengths and your mind. It will hide you from others. This is for further techniques.

Self-harmonizing-

This is a sensory technique. First, get into a meditative position. Feel yourself in your gut. Pull towards your stomach to minimize the self. Imagine an image of yourself condensed within yourself. Imagine it shrinking to your gut. Condense yourself by feeling you in yourself. This is to minimize presence.

Hand gestures-

There are multiple hand gestures to manipulate your bio magnetic field. One way is hiding presences, other movements include the tai chi orb, isolation movement, discharging, and then a Zen circle.

To use the tai chi orb, use cross streaming to charge up, then hold one hand at the center of the chest and the other below it palms facing inward to each other. Curve your hands and make them move away from each other about two inches away and then go back, do this several times to feel your chi connecting.

Next is an isolation movement. Put your hands out palms facing outward. Next, move both hands in a three-foot line downwards, then up in a 2-foot line, then down in a one-foot line, and then push out away from yourself. This is an isolation technique.

To discharge, use the cross-stream technique to charge up, then move one hand across your other arm, this should discharge your biofield.

To do a Zen circle, start with one hand up at your forehead, and the other at your stomach then make them move in a large circle, each hand in the opposite direction, when you get to the center of the body move your hands in towards each other. Do this slow for a biosphere drag. It is good to center the self before doing this.

Pathway Creation

This is a building block for other techniques. Understanding this technique is very important. Practicing this technique will allow greater usage later. Use this on multiple parts of the body, to allow further mastery of this.

Channeling-

This is a body technique. We are a simultaneous charge that builds up in the body. We can create a pathway to dump a charge or to cleanse ourselves. To create this pathway, flex the bicep, release and flex the forearm, then release and flex the hand. Speed up fluctuation, like the following: (1 2   3), (1   2   3), (1 2 3), (123).

Once you push to (123) all after that is you vibrating your arm. Now vibrate your arm and push with sequence.

That is how you channel energy.

Now channel backward, starting from hand to forearm to bicep. This pattern is a draw.

You can channel at different parts of the body, like the leg, torso, chest, or head. For example, if you channel your jaw, cheek, then ear muscles it will unlock your brain frequency. This may require a little bit of practice, but when you feel it, it will be like a vibration in the brain. This will unlock your neuroplasticity, and muscle memory. This is the organization of your muscles. To get a clearer view, you are only channeling in one direction, but it is the frequency in which you restart the process to push your energy further.

Remember you are a field, and when channeling these vibrations you can channel past your own field, creating yourself into a pathway. You aren't losing any energy, you are simply creating a pathway for energy to travel on.

Micro Sensory

The goal is tuning your senses to the smallest variables possible. The physical body can only pick up at a certain level, so we push the boundaries of that level by tunning in our focus onto almost untraceable variables, and enhancing that with focus, strengthening the edges of our perception.

Pinpoint sensory-

This is a sensory technique. First, feel your hand and your foot opposite of each other simultaneously, now switch sides. Concentrate on only those parts.

Now feel your feet touching the floor. Concentrate on your feet only. Feel the vibration of the body concentrated in the feet only. This hides your vibration. Now try it with other points of the body, concentrating on the feeling of touch.

Next is pinpoint sensory. Touch your hand with your finger, then feel that spot without the finger. Now feel parts of the body without touching anything. This exercises your skin sensitivity.

If you can't feel parts of your body, then touch that point and feel that point to exercise it. Also dragging the feeling to points of the body allows it to heal the other parts. This allows the reconnection of your nervous system.

Some points can change your habits. For example, if you put your thumb on the roof of your mouth, and feel just the thumb, you can curb hunger.

Redundancy-

This is a layered sensory technique. Understand that tuning your focus to specific spots creates redundancy in the system. One way to create redundancy is by hyper-focusing on a spot, which can be done by feeling specifically one spot while ignoring the rest of the body's feelings. The simultaneous systems in the body naturally create multiple fields acting at once. Further techniques will allow the focus on specific systems while utilizing them with other systems, creating redundancy.

Signal hand-

This is a sensory technique. Feel the upper palm between the pointer and the middle finger. Touch this part of the hand with your other hand, then touch the part between your pinky and ring finger. Touch these parts then feel these parts without your hand. Feel from one part to the other back and forth as fast as possible. Once you establish this connection use channeling to push through the charge at the same time as feeling them. Shape your hand into a V between your middle and ring finger when channeling. This form is the same way an antenna works. This will be used further with other techniques.

Listening hand-

This is a passive sensory technique. First, get into a meditative position. Hold your hand out in front of you and relax your hand. Listen to the skin on your hand, now make your hand an extension of your listening, rather than listening to it, listen with it. Start the process of meditation and focus on listening with your hand. This is the listening palm, which can be paired with feeling later with specific uses. Practice going into listening form without meditation. The hand is the best place to start, however, you can do this with other parts of the skin. This technique is used further later.

Chi Charging

This is a powerful way to build chi, both yin, and yang. With central condensing, one can learn to increase their spirit pressure by how much chi they can hold, in turn, this technique allows for advanced usage of chi. Practice makes perfect.

Heavy concentration breathing-

This is a breathing technique. Inhale through the nose, and exhale out the nose, this is to build up dark chi. Concentrate on the breath while breathing, and go about your day breathing through your nose, while thinking about it. After doing this for some time, breathe in through your nose deeply and let out a large exhale through your mouth. Do this till the body releases all the dark chi you built up. You can feel the dark chi build in your brow. After exhaling, this should relax you tremendously. Now try inhaling through your mouth while thinking about it and exhaling through your mouth while thinking about it. This is light chi build-up. You may feel the build up in the chin. To end inhale through the mouth deeply and exhale through the nose to burn off light chi. You can also try this by inhaling through the mouth and exhaling through the nose or inhaling through the nose and exhaling through the mouth. Every version requires a cooldown when exiting the cycle. Whichever of the four versions you use, note the body's feeling when you end the cycle. The one that made you feel the best is your version of chi usage. More on this later.

Emotional Control

Control over emotion is best done before you get emotional. Practicing reflection helps stabilize our emotions and enhance our demeanor. Prevented maintenance only works if you do it, so take the time to learn control, by abolishing hatred, and quelling anger. We can have irrational fear reactions, as well as irrational anger, sadness, love, and joy. Learn to rationalize your emotions, and you will find truth in your reactions.

Obtaining Serenity-

This is an emotional technique. Emotion is a reaction; however, we can trick reaction by creating the byproduct of the reaction without the reactant being there. This is a form of emotional control. First, you will want to establish a base aspect, which is like valor or calmness. To gain a base is to be that base or have done that base. The base is only as strong as you have created it to be through action. First, we start by opening ourselves up to the truth.

Get into a meditative position and focus on yourself. Surrender not to a moment but surrender to the whole of moments that you created in life. What are you in life? Have you done enough, just starting, doing too much? What is the balance of your sin? Of your hatred? Surender to these things and feel the whole of the self. This is a way to gauge yourself and see what needs to be worked on. Do not deny yourself, that blocks the path, be truthful about yourself. If you cannot see your truth, who will? You open yourself to weakness and defeat yourself before someone defeats you. Try to do things like, I do not hate, I hope they get better, to want them to become better or even to be happy. If you are not clear enough, you must engage to clear yourself.

True serenity can only be obtained by surrendering to the truth of the self. Try not to gauge yourself to others, you are your worst enemy. Truth is not always easy, but not always bad. Also, be satisfied with your truth. It is what you created and what you are worthy of. If you're not satisfied, then change it. Only you can do that.

Base aspects-

This is an emotional technique. This technique allows a base for emotional channeling. There are multiple bases you can use. The bases we will cover are neutral, calm, serious, and righteous. There are other bases good and bad, such as hope, melancholy, boredom, satisfaction, and contentment. These are natural bases we can go through, and a similar technique can be done to utilize these bases but will always be accessed from another viewpoint. We will focus on the ones that utilize emotions best.

Neutral is a feelingless base. Get into a meditative position, and focus on nothing, neutral means you are neutral to all emotions, and all other bases. You're just matter. Move your hands slowly from hips to your shoulders, and feel yourself drag what is yours aside, this is a way to cleanse the self. You can also walk forward and feel the drag of yourself, cleansing you into your base matter. This will be used further later.

Calm can be achieved physically. First, use the meditative breathing technique, focusing on the exhale on top of the pallet. Feel your anxiety leave the body, what is naturally leftover is calm. You can use this with anger, and other emotions to calm the self. Using this technique and the neutral technique together also works.

Seriousness varies on the user. The truth of your discipline is what you can conjure. Use your strictness of yourself as an example. In martial arts, it is the discipline that allows one to become the machine one makes. Use this with no joking around you. Calm or neutralize the self, then conjure your "I mean business" feeling, or the deep-in-work feeling, the feeling that gets you there, not the result, but the process of work.

Righteousness is just righteous in its own right. This one is about holding honor and truth. Use your honor and justice together and you conjure righteousness. Use this after you use the neutral or calm technique, then focus on your honor. Once you establish honor, you can add your discipline to this. Righteousness is a weapon version, and seriousness is the tool version. Simply add justice, and or focus to obtain either base.

As long as you can describe the base, you can find it. Each base will always feel different to the user, no user is the same, however, there is a similarity to all and a limit. The limit for the most part is you and your experiences, as well as our matters limits.

Emotional movement-

This is an emotional body technique. When you get angry, a set of muscles activates, causing intensity in the body, tightness in the throat, and other physical movements based on anger. Without being angry, tighten those muscles and tighten the inner throat. When doing this use a channeling technique from the arm to the palm. Anger intensifies channeling; however, it is tricking the body into being angry rather than being angry. Add anger to an emotional aspect, you can unlock serious anger or righteous anger.

When you get sad, glands activate and can cause a spiral of emotion. To trick the body into sorrow, tighten the outside of the neck, pull in on the stomach, and relax the orbicularis oculi, which is the muscle on top of the cheek and below the eye. This is how you trick the body into sorrow. Again, do this with a base to empower your chi. You will notice when using tai chi this emotional stance is stronger with inner instinct. Follow the movement of the emotions through your instinct, follow your inner chi.

When you get happy, you tighten the orbicularis oculi and push upwards on the skin. Do this to trick the body into happiness. Use this with the bases above, you may find many combos there like elated or successful.

Love is usually just a reaction. To trick the body into love, relax the entirety of the inner throat and jaw. These gives extremes with bases. If you have trouble relaxing the middle inner throat, place your fingers on the throat and relax the throat, this goes with the anybody point relaxation technique. Choose your reactions wisely.

Unlocking The Innate Mind

This unlocks patterns that are passively you. These techniques further unlock possibilities and help you learn more about yourself. These are based on your preset strengths.

Combo sensory-

This is a sensory method technique. Your body is fully connected (all connected) and so are your senses through simultaneous systems. Tuning in this sense requires material items. You will need a clear quartz crystal pendulum. This is required to see the movements of people's energy.

First, dip the crystal alongside a willing subject's hand 3 times. You are focusing on the subject's body energy. Move the pendulum one inch above the subject's palm, holding the chain straight, and move it up the arm. You will feel a slight tug when you encounter their energy path. Movements can determine numbness in the hand, skin conditions, arthritis, and other such integumentary nervous damage. After you trace their hand energy, use the blinking technique with a light to see their hand outline. If your third eye is awakened, you should be able to see their movements. Remember it is like listening and it is their movements and truth. Sometimes people, especially children, have guardians that will interact with your third eye, especially if you have a third eye awakened and do the 5-blink technique. You can use the blinking technique against the sun to get a better aura view with the physical eye. This technique takes practice and time, patience, and visual listening, and can be utilized in multiple ways, as we will use later. This is exercising the eye-touch combo sensory in your mind.

Other combos must be unlocked in other ways. If you'd like to utilize other combo senses, practice smelling different smells, smelling what's around you from your location, you can go further by using the tongue and nose together may already know what things taste and smell like. Even using smell to hone in on specific smells or smaller trails of smell. You can tune your ears and skin together to practice telecommunication. Every aspect of our DNA makes this combo based on heritage, race, and sex; the differentials create differentials in ways to telecommunicate. Some mountain people in thinner air seem to be louder, while some in the humid areas tend to speak more with images in the humidity, more projector-type minds. Some families can project together to create in flow, or to create a telepathic circle.

This comes with time and experimentation, however is not dangerous to the user. Make sure you cleanse your space before you perform, and always allow plants to be within the home, especially in what you would consider haunted areas, this seems to absorb their wavelengths, trees do this especially.

Unlocking ferocity-

This is a body instinct technique. First, cross-stream and get charged. Have a prepared physical task to channel your ferocity, like swimming, running, climbing, or along those lines. Take your hand and place it spread across the middle of your head. Pull upwards from the thumb to the pointer, to center, and pull up.

Next, perform a task and allow it to open up your mind which should engage all senses and body movement simultaneously. You may move through the water faster, open up your sprint, gauge jumps and sticking landings, and things like this flow on a natural bond. This is used further to unlock instinct when called upon regularly. There is always a cooldown on the first use. Meaning you will feel brain pain after a task. This is used later.

Memory Sequence-

This is a memory technique. First gather some items, something you can see, something you can taste, something you can smell, and something you do like putting on a glove. Next, think of a phrase and something that reflects emotion. Finally do all the tasks, taste, smell, feel, and say the phrase will do it. Do this with someone else as a control. Next, wait 15 minutes, what do you remember first? Next, wait a couple of hours, and see what you remember first. You can do this at length from days to a week. Whatever you remember first is the primary sense for short-term memory. Whatever you remember later, the further the better, is your sense that holds your long-term memory. Doing this will determine how you remember.

You can even pull up memories better once you unlock what your primary form of remembering is. For example, how you felt, how it felt, textures, the color of objects leading to what surrounded it, the sound of something, and even numbers, dates, and so forth. You'll find that you will start to unlock memories based on specific details.

Bloodline techniques-

These are passive techniques. They can range from your chi form, to your natural dream perspective, to your natural combo sensory techniques, and also to your natural telecommunication perspective. Understanding chi forms are under chi mage, the first style. Explore this to understand the natural alignment of your chi, which can range from elemental prowess to abstract connections. Your natural dream can range from Deja Vu dreams to spiritual dreams, and even deeper insight dreams, depending on what you are sensitive to, or what you've been exposed to. Combo sensory varies based on your strongest senses, and how you use your third eye, which can vary from person to person. Telecommunication can be different from echo communication, projector sight, and Mushi share technique to a range of other things, every person is different, and is usually based on heritage and bloodline, just like the other three.

Cleansing Shi

It is important to have a cleansed space to work in, however, you must be prepared to cleanse your space. Therefore, you must have these other techniques down before you cleanse, just in case you have some encounters.

Cleansing-

It is important to cleanse a space before you practice. Using sound bowls helps cleanse the wavelengths in an area. Penetrating the wavelengths in an area, with sound, cleanses the area for practice. Another way to cleanse the area is a calm blue flame. The intensity of the fire cleanses spaces, and while a torch works, a calm blue flame penetrates the wavelengths of the earth. Use butane sprayed into a shot glass, or for example ax spray to create a calm blue flame. The subtle intensity penetrates the wavelength of the area. Incense works as well to cleanse the area. It is important to know how to cleanse as well as how to defend from outer forces.

The practice of bowing to the sun is simply a practice of grounding and allowing the earth's rotation to naturally cleanse the self. Therefore, praying for three hours a day is used, however excessive, it is a practice of grounding the body of any wavelengths that are not of the body. Understanding how to use the earth requires time, and that is why it is done for long periods. While this is a great technique, it does not have to be done often only when you feel another presence is afflicting you. Remember that your heart is constantly beating, and the blood's magnetism is constantly rotating in you, causing a constant rotating field, which cleanses itself, so therefore, it is possible to cleanse from spiritual marks, (ghost marks) just by existing. You basically absorb them. Remember you are life, and they do not exist anymore, meaning you will always win against the undead.

There are three forms of grounding. One is to the earth, which grounds higher magnetic wavelengths that can be caused by using wands or other forms of tech within the practice. being touched also makes this effect that can be grounded when done. Parasitic entities or hauntings can be recycled through trees. Grounding through trees is effective to get rid of overactive wavelengths within the body. Your body produces a default of what its matter is, so grounding is good to get rid of excess energy. Grounding to metal gets rid of electrical charge build up in the body as well. Rubber can be used as a medium between you and the charge. Rubber mouthpieces can be used to ground built-up charges in the teeth. To do this, put the rubber mouthpiece in your mouth and touch the ground with the mouthpiece while in your mouth. This will draw the charge that can be caught in wisdom teeth, holes in the mouth, or even ear issues.

Always be cautious, and make your house your space, don't let other things dictate your space. More information on this will be given further.

Spiritual tuning-

This is a sensory technique. The spiritual is just the magnetism of the earth, going through matter and causing a drag, creating (indoors) a bluish-gray hue. There are multiple types of remnants from the earth, like ley lines and other things. This will be covered later. We have our fields, so to touch the field around us takes some practice.

Get into a meditative pose and quiet your energy. You can do this with relaxation. Then reach your hand out and tap your finger as if taping the top of the water. You should feel a tap, maybe a ripple, or a dip, perhaps even a drag. Depending on your response depends on your next attempt. If you feel a tap, use your whole hand then push through the tap. If you feel a ripple, use your finger again and leave it in the ripple, once you feel the ripple allow your hand to move through the entrance and feel the ripple around your hand. If you feel a dip, dip again and snake your hand into the dip as if diving. If you feel a drag, touch with all your fingertips, once you do this rip through as if scratching. Next just go through. If you feel the tap-hold hands to your side and walk through the tap all at once. if you feel a ripple allow yourself to walk through the ripple point. Feel the ripple move across your body. If you feel a dip, dive through the dip point. Feel yourself emerge. If you feel the drag, use the breaststroke to tear through the feeling. Walk forward while doing hand motions. If you cannot get through, station an anchor point, using it as a reference for an entrance, like a doorway.

Spiritual reveal-

This is a sensory technique. Place your hand on your other hand's fingertips. Pull your hand from your fingertips to your wrist. As you pull, pull your magnetism back with your hand. Feel your revealed hand as you pull back your magnetism. It should react with the magnetic sphere of the earth telling you. When doing this understand that your results may not be as you might expect. Usually, the result is in an elemental form. Know that the elements of the periodic table and their movements are everything. Another way to do this is to push your hands forward while channeling backward. This can also be used as a cleansing. Pulling back on the hand with muscle while pushing forward on the skin allows a cleanse as well, allowing your hand to be filled with a feeling. This can also be a reveal if focused on that.

Dream Law

There are some rules to follow before you start on your journey of lucid dreaming. First, you are the anchor of your dream, you can always go back to the self, and your body generates the dream, so you cannot leave your body. You can project your mind outside of the self, however, there are some steps to do this. Remember you are your body, not your energy, the body produces the energy. So, when dreaming you are the anchor.

Abstract contrast-

It is important to recognize when others are with you in the dream and when they are not. It is important to recognize entities and spirits as well. We don't usually dream at their frequency, but they can interface with you. Abstract contrast is recognizing something that is not you with you. It is recognizing visitation, this can happen in many ways but when you start to lucid dream, dream walk, or meditate you open the possibilities of visitation.

Usually, the visitation is positive. Alien visitation only happens when they are physically there, same with evil spirits, they must be there. Think of it like wild animals, you don't always see them or rarely see them, and if you want to see one you usually must travel to its territory. Therefore, when dreaming, these negative entities are only where they are. Visitation of greater spirits or guardians can happen if they are there waiting for you to wake up, usually through enlightenment, or successful meditation. Dream walkers may sense the presence of other living beings, or other entities guarding certain places. To learn dream walking and places to go, look under Dream walker.

Differentials-

Abstract contrast is about recognizing others, differentials are about recognizing the environment. Recognizing the difference between you and the environment allows you to see the order in which it is constructed, some environments are not the same as ours and are constructed outside the laws of physics. Understanding that if it exists it has an order. This can also enhance your dreams by being more aware of the dreamscape, liking feeling grass, or the sun on your skin in a dream environment brings out a manifestation of your detail, which in turn can also tell you what you need.

Literal dreams-

These dreams are Deja Vu. The closer the dream is to real the more likely it can be seen in real-time. Usually, the dreams are 5 to 15 seconds long, always in first person, and usually 3 weeks ahead of time. These are DeJa'Vu and come with a feeling. When you catch a DeJa'Vu it works as a sense of time, allowing further dreams to be detected, and sometimes even greater DeJa'Vu that resonate with other beings of prediction or major events seen throughout time. These are rare however when tuned into, can be a huge asset.

Sorcery Mechanics

Sorcery is the play with energies around you, created by outside sources. Sensory is a huge way of tuning into sorcery. These are the basic mechanics when it comes to sorcery.

The 6 movements-

This is a sensory technique. This uses the 6 usable movements in the body that we can use: heat, light, electricity, magnetism, sound, and vibration. To sense these properties, you must expose yourself to these movements.

We have been at 98 degrees all our lives. We create heat within our bodies. The consistency of our body's temperature creates a differential from everything else. We are 98 degrees, and everything is not necessarily the same. Notice the differentials between you and the environment around you, from the air to any item you can think of. This contrast is a unique sensation that is used with some styles. This is a sensory technique used later.

Light creates heat, and not all light feels the same. Turn on a light and feel the light's heat. This is a way of sensing light; another way is to understand what type of light it is and how it's moving. Some light bounce, and some move in straight pathways, regardless a light always creates a Luxon in a particle atmosphere. The color of light moves at different wavelength frequencies, so you can feel the difference between purple light and red light. More on this later.

Exposing the self to electricity can be dangerous. One way to safely feel electricity is to get a plasma orb. Understanding the properties of electricity is very important in its use and can be created in the body if the user knows how. The intensity of electricity will not be the same due to the differentials in the matter however can be achieved at a specific level. More on how electricity works later.

Magnetism can be sensed when using magnets with each other. To sense the body's magnetism, you need to have 4 to 6 magnets, pointing their similar poles inward, to create a magnetic push. This push allows the body to sense the pole differentials in the blood. This technique is mostly sensory awareness.

Sound is already somewhat mystical. A part of your body can read the wavelengths and vibrations in the air, in the ear. Utilizing the ear for listening is probably the most efficient technique.

Vibrations in air can be sensed, and so can vibration through the ground and objects. This is harder to sense but exposing yourself to vibration allows the sensory to tune in.

The most important thing to remember is that our senses can be tuned in, but to tune them in requires understanding and awareness. Keep an open mind.

U tuning-

The planet is in constant motion on a grand scale. We are not attuned to its movement. Nor are we tuned to its magnetic sphere or its gravity. However, we are naturally tuned involuntarily, not necessarily aware of it. We can tune ourselves into time as well, as well as the sun and other outside sources.

To tune into the earth, you must understand that we rotate about 460 meters per second at the equator in space. This suggests we have a drag through our rotation. Get into a meditative state and use the free flow technique. While feeling free flow, feel the drag of the earth. Once you confirm your relativity you can feel the drag of the earth, this is better done outside.

Once you tune in to the earth's speed now you can tune into the earth's magnetic sphere. Use the free flow technique then raise your hands slowly from your sides to your shoulders. You should feel your drag through the magnetic sphere. Understand that energy comes in threes, so you may feel three layers of drag. The core is 1802 miles deep, and the magnetism of the core goes through all 1802 miles at the poles and encompasses us into its reverberation of the magnetic sphere.

Gravity can be sensed in the ear. We have a base level of sensory sensitivity for gravity, however sometimes when we are a little bigger our bodies give into complacency, so we don't feel so miserable. Don't allow this, feel your gravity, and you will be miserable, which will help you burn weight. Some people might be already quite attuned to our gravity.

Time is easier to tune into. Time is always the same variables are always constant, however, how much you can fit into one second is not constant and variable. Throw a punch, most of us pay attention to the beginning, the middle, and the end, throw, hit, retraction. Now throw a punch at the same speed and feel throw, extension, hit, retraction, extend. In other words, feel the full variables during the punch and you can tune into milliseconds. Adding a rotation to the punch also allows more variables to track, therefore tuning in the punch in milliseconds more naturally.

Another way to tune into time is through the center rotation of the sun. Once you get a DeJa'Vu dream, which is always first person, about a 30-second clip, and 3 weeks ahead, you can sense when it's happening, almost as if you can sense time. Once you get a DeJa'Vu time dream, you can recognize the feeling of DeJa'Vu. The more you recognize, the smaller the 30-second gap gets. The more control you have the less you see. However, it is just the amount you see that is less, down to uncountable variables like 3 seconds long. Once you get tuned in you can even sense DeJa'Vu on a grand scale.

Sorcery

This is a material technique. Understand that feeling comes from all things and your interactions. The source still has a pattern that we can feel. Using materials like stones, and metals, we can get reactions with these specific frequencies. Remember that your reaction is of two ways, harm or heal, or a mixture of both. but the reaction is always further to what you are using. Some stones are good for cleansing the body, like dragon bloodstones, or for other uses. Metals are also used like this. The most basic metals with reaction are gold, silver, copper, and iron. We can also get different feelings with different colored lights.

We can use technological systems as sources of energy. We can use these pathways created by material to create pathways with which we can interact. Further the study of technology with the mystic arts later. Understanding technology is understanding nature, and in all is just the basics of how reality works. Don't be afraid to accept technology in life, however knowing it can be a tool of human purpose. Use basic tech and the way it works to manifest a tool for your sorcery, or in other words wands. Channeling through an object pushes electricity, and later can be used to manipulate movements of the elements and so forth. Understanding what you can use is what makes this so worthwhile. To understand a wand is to understand all things, it's like a graduation gift. If you read through this and learn your way, the next step is using equipment and creating it.

Eternal Knowledge

The 8-

This is a knowledge technique. The first rotation can be used to hold information other than with the 4 phases, and 4 movements. It can be used to hold the body's anatomy, a physical process of life, and even an emotional process that was used by the buddha, the 8 divine truths. While there are many aspects in which you can use the 8, the focus is on the anatomical information the 8 and 16 hold together, using them can help you understand and access more of the body. Also understanding the aspect of the elements is by understanding their literal properties. More on this later.

House families-

This is a knowledge technique. This focus is on families. The third family square is all on the physical recycling process. This process is used in the body, represented by the systems of recycling in the body, as well as a system of emotional recycling, and recycling in our biosphere. The fourth square is represented by the things that can grow. This is a family of houses of energy. Each line is a combo between the two energies, giving a house line. Plasma to organic is life energy, or the energy of the nervous system, and the reaction of the nervous system. Plasma to mineral/crystal is the lifeblood, like sap, skin or blood, the absorbers of energy. Crystal to atmosphere creates the salt crystal, or the chrysalis, the saltwater environment. Atmosphere to organic is the process and the reaction of oxygen, or oxidation. Organic to Crystal is the power of the structure, from the mineral build-up to the structure of the tree, this is called the house of amber. This is a long house and has more of a twin structure than one house altogether. The other house is from plasma to atmosphere, giving us sunlight, or the reaction of a plasma's aura going through a particle atmosphere generating the Luxon, both a process of sunlight. These are 6 houses that each come with energy.

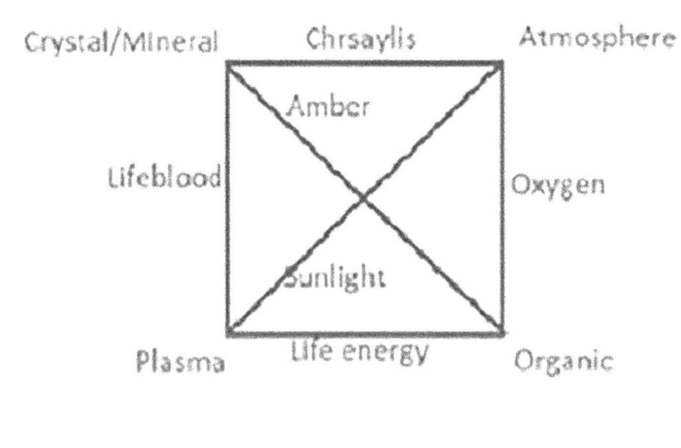

Styles

There are 99 styles in this book that can mix and match with each other to make your style. At the end of the book, there are pages for your notes, so you can start creating your spells.

Most of the styles are sorted by their name. Wizard is the name of the practitioners. Sorcerers use a source of energy outside of the body and use their bodies to make pathways for energy. Mancers manifest from themselves, by putting the body into a specific state or using a specific state. Mages use eternal movements and movements of the body to affect the area. benders can bend the environment to them or shape it another way. Sages follow the art of healing.

Healing

Healing is in the interest of survival; you cannot heal that which is already healed. This is part of the mindset of healing. Healing is also a source of white necromancy, which is the idea to preserve what already exists. Healing can also take place by seeking what causes issues, allowing users to dive into a world of their personal qualities, or their own experience to heal in many ways. Healing can also come from the ability to control your states of emotions and to avoid the feeling of denial. Remember the hardest part is navigating through yourself is finding the perspective that isn't yours yet. Healers use the tools of how and why to find and fix the problem. Always be aware, you cannot heal the dead, for the undead cannot heal. These are just a few aspects of healing. Part of the dark side is in healing, that life unchecked by death has no enemy, inviting the creation of selfish emotions as a side effect of long-lasting life. Fill life with purpose, knowledge, and guidance and you will find everlasting life. Remember the body will always seek harmony with itself.

Spirit

The spirit is the raw energy of how you navigate through life. both in our actions, and reactions. Learning the spirit is a personal journey, like our chi, our emotions, and our experiences which all shape the spirit.

Chi mage

Overview: unlock the power of your raw chi, to understand your techniques and what you can use strongest. This will set you up for further styles.

Techniques used: Chi charging, Mindscape building

Knowledge: Understanding Chi:

Chi is used for describing the energy that is created in the body during the breath. However, there are multiple ways to understand chi. One is the reaction of the breath, which is used in this case with concentration breathing. Another is your inner instinct flow, which is used elsewhere, and the final is the dark and light inner chi your body makes through its complexities. Unlocking inner chi is like seeing the complexity of your personality etched in the form of the elements. There are two types of chis, dark and light chi. While there are dark and light reactions there are also dark and dark as well as light and light reactions. The light and the dark are easy ways to see the complexity of what it is. To see into the light and dark chis and understand their further complexities is the goal of being a chi mage.

Spells: building chi- To build up light chi breathe in through the mouth and exhale through the mouth. Concentrate on the breath leaving and touching the top of your pallet. Do this for a minute, and you will start to build light chi naturally. breathe normally for a minute to cleanse the self. To build up dark chi breathe in through the nose and exhale through the nose while holding your brow tight. This will build up dark chi, do this for a minute, then breath normal for a minute to balance the self out again.

Using chi- next, build up light chi, and feel the light flow through the body, not just your mind. Feel the reaction taking place and feel the light chi. Next channel while building chi, channel from your arm down and feel the light chi, moving the concentration of light chi around the body by focusing on other parts of the body. Cool down by breathing normally and doing the same thing while building dark chi. You can now call on dark or light chi, which means all you have to do is feel the chi state to be in it, this will react with whatever chi state you are physically holding, being a two-part reaction.

Reactions- There are 8 types of reactions. First, there is the chi stance, which is light or dark heavy concentration breathing. Next is using a chi with your chi stance, like pushing light through your light chi stance, or pulling causes a reaction, each reaction is different, and some reactions may not happen because it is unknown to you. These are the 8 reactions:

Light stance while pulling light

Light stance while pushing light

Light stance while pulling dark

Light stance while pushing dark

Dark stance while pulling dark

Dark stance while pushing dark

Dark stance while pulling light

Dark stance while pushing light

To pull use reverse channeling (in basics), and use the mind's eye technique, or open third eye technique to see your movements. Do these 8 reactions and see the movements of your chi. This will give you an idea of what you are meant for.

Advanced: It is best to write down the 8 forms and your findings. These findings will always be represented as a movement of the 8 elements, or the elements. Sometimes you might find abstract abilities, other times none at all. Take the stance that suits you best, which is usually the one with the highest reactions. Use these as a base for what you might strive in. As you go through the book you will find styles that suit your natural chi type.

Emomancer

Overview: inducing the body into emotional states

Techniques: Emotional control

Knowledge: Understanding emotion:

There are four basic emotional responses, sorrow, love, joy, and anger. Each one sets off body reactions. Learning these reactions allows us to use emotion outside of response. Each of the body's responses responds differently with energy. There are other emotions, what makes these so special is each can be set off immediately, whereas some may have a delay or only after-the-fact responses. Regardless, these have strong body responses that can be manipulated.

Spells: Sorrow- Sorrow is an inward movement, caused by turmoil in the inner self, which causes an inward movement. To induce sorrow, use your outer neck muscles to pull down on the throat, and pull inward on the stomach, while loosening the orbicularis oculi, just under the eye. This induces sorrow, which can be used to help charge the body.

Love- Love is a reaction of its own that can fill you with energy. Love is as varied as people; it will always be different from person to person. The goal is not to cause a reaction in people but within the self. Love without sexual desire is pure love, which you can also feel with gratitude. When using the following technique use it with gratitude for existence, the planet, and life. Place three fingers along the center of the throat spaced along the center. Tighten the throat, then feel these spots and relax the inner throat starting from the center finger traveling up and down to the other fingers, entirely and simultaneously. This will unlock love.

Joy- Joy is uplifting and relaxing at the same time. Tighten your fists then release and hold the release, then tighten your body while releasing. Also relaxing then tightening the throat and the orbicularis oculi for a similar result. Some reactions can happen depending on your state of being, meaning you can have sorrow for feeling happy or loved. Joy can be used for its release of energy.

Anger- Anger is intense, and can amplify energy. Tighten your body to feel anger, for intense anger, focus on tightening your chest and your lower jaw and throat muscles. Anger will focus your attention making you single- minded so targeting something to focus on can help, you don't have to be angry at the target for this to work.

Advanced: Use emotions accordingly to work out stressful problems, also some emotions like love can be used with a partner. Remember matter is what we are, we are programmed to react in specific ways, and there is no taboo in using emotion. It is there for your use and you can use it any way you want. If we were not meant to feel it we wouldn't have organs that produce the feeling anyway.

Love has its place for filling the body with energy. Sorrow can be used to harness the energy, anger can be used to amplify that energy, and joy can be used to release it. You can use these techniques to strengthen multiple styles.

Memory Mancer

Overview: utilizes the ability to recall moments in time.

Techniques: Unlocking the innate mind, Boundary understanding

Knowledge: Memory:

Memory is based on our senses reacting with the physical world. Memory is made up of senses, movements, and reactions. Focusing on listening to a moment helps strengthen the passive ability to remember a moment. As children, we start to develop memory based on the molecular level of absorption, which takes years to develop, meaning we are not able to hold memory till we are at the right age, around 3 to 5. However, deeper memories when described can be remembered based on the fact we were there, and we are listening as children. Time is a constant, and we are flowing through that constant, and memory is based on moments through time.

Spells: Tapping memory- We remember moments in detail, usually recalling entire moments through a single detail. This detail is usually based on how you remember. Some may remember the color of an object, the feeling of an object, the smell of something, the sound of something, or even the emotion at the time. Find your detail to unlock memory.

Full body memory- Your body is always present in memory, even if it was of something else, the body is what is recording that moment. We can recall moments in time better when we incorporate the full body. We can also create stronger memories by incorporating the entire body into a situation. Take a moment to feel your whole body, remember that feeling. Do an activity while feeling your whole body. Then recall what you just did, and you will recall the entirety of the memory as if you were flowing with time.

Intensify moments- To intensify memory you use the whole body plus listening to your senses while doing an activity. You start to incorporate multiple parts of the brain for this memory. Remembering all senses all together at once strengthens a moment of memory.

Advanced: Meditation can help focus the senses by focusing on one sense while meditating. To understand further memory, it is good to know the structure of the brain and its sequence of operation, to fully understand memory. Remember our memory is based on the brain's structure. This can help organize the self-further.

Healer

Healing is about balancing the body, and about maintaining specific states of health.

Channel Sage

Overview: focuses on channeled healing

Technique: Pathway creation, Eternal knowledge

Knowledge: white necromancy:

White necromancy is the idea of the preservation of life, to keep one alive beyond death. To preserve we must preserve our structure, by maintaining its function, which means maintaining PH, cellular degeneration, and structural integrity. To do this we must eat right to maintain a balanced ph. Enlightenment allows neuroplasticity as well as cellular regeneration, which allows cells to divide with positive energy. Staying in one piece makes it easier to maintain structure, as well as keep structural integrity, which can reduce problems in the future. Healing is based on your systems trying to maintain your optimum state of health. These following techniques are for activating your systems when you get hurt, allowing an acceleration in healing due to your involvement with your healing, causing redundancy in the signal which strengthens the process. The more you know the easier it is to heal. Understanding the hidden systems is very important, this will accelerate your healing like you're healing with reserved energy. by creating these physical pathways of consciousness, you cause redundancy which backs up your back up.

Spells: Channeling the 8- This is using the basic channel technique with the knowledge of the eight elements. When you push the octagon, you activate all systems which are located in the body. It is like making a neural connection with your systems, just knowing the chakra systems in the body allows you to feel all those systems in the body. Without this you can still activate the systems with basic channeling, however, knowing and focusing on other systems we don't feel allow greater results.

Rune channel- The 192-pointed star naturally holds energy, or movements, so using this with channeling and visual channeling naturally empowers channeling. Using a bigger version allows for greater meditative use, as well as greater visual channeling. The rune can also gather energies that don't belong in the body, like possession, disease, and other types of movements that aren't typical from the physical source. After use, it is good to cleanse the image with light.

All together- You can use the 192-pointed stars with the knowledge of the 16 systems and channeling to further your ability to heal. Focusing on the 4 things that grow allows you to tap into the 6 houses. These houses of energy are powerful tools for cleansing and work best when meditating and channeling.

Advanced: To further your scope it is good to focus on various ways to channel, using things like the brain frequency technique, or full body channel, as well as furthering knowledge of anatomy.

Zen Sage

Overview: focuses on nerve healing

Technique: Qi connections

Knowledge: Connections

The body is like an electrical system. When a switch is off, there is no pathway for the electricity to flow, if it is on it will flow, and be on instantly. The nervous system works like this as well, it also can work like a load. A load is like a light bulb or a motor. When the connection is made, they turn on, so when we complete the circuit, the light bulb gets brighter and becomes like a load. This is when you reach Zen, you complete the circuit, and your brain turns into a load. When we read the body, we are looking for disruptions in the circuit, and a connection in the body to make a load. It is good to have your third eye active before attempting these spells. These spells also require that you have a clear quartz crystal pendant.

Spells:

Body trace- to trace the body use the pendant and dip it past your or someone else's hand three times, for cleansing and connection. Use the pendant to follow the body's energy, created by blood flow and nervous connection. Follow the body with the pendant and notice that the pendant will lean towards the path of movement. Where there is no movement, you have an ignored spot. Ignored spots usually cause a redirection of movement, and can even cause puddling, meaning the pendant will flow in a circle. Use the next spell to heal ignored or puddling spots.

Nerve connects- You can use light as a brush for the nervous system, or your hands. Regardless of what you choose, channel through your hand or light outward and pull from around the ignored spot through it to reconnect the spot to the nervous system. Puddles can be massaged out or redirected with channeling or pulled on with your energy brush to complete the circuit. Use the next spell once you reconnect systems, to find their Zen pose.

Zen drop- To find the Zen pose, first clear your systems by channeling. Next is to find the path of less resistance. Maneuver the hands in a way that allows connection to each other. When they have connected the energy, when traced, will have no movement. They should be sitting straight, and their hands connected in their Zen pose which is the body's connection to create a load within them. This pose causes the brain to act as a load, creating focus. The position that generates the most focus in the brain is the Zen pose. When the circuit is complete the focus is made in the brain. Detecting these loads is done in the hands, you will have no movement of the crystal if they are in a loading state. It will be clear and have a drop, meaning no movement. Moving the hands into different positions is key for finding the drop. When the circuit in the hands is a complete circuit, you will find the drop.

Advanced: Every zen pose is different for every individual. Damaged structures in the arms will cause zen poses to flow based on that physical impairment or injury. A correct zen pose can have extreme reactions to healing. These techniques can be paired with massage therapy, reiki, and acupuncture.

Harmonizer

Overview: focuses on balance

Technique: Hidden techniques

Knowledge: balance:

Life is an energetic positive. Nothing is physical space; something is a positive. Planets and stars are super energetic positives, and life is energetic positives. We are a singularity, and when we harmonize, we do so within our relativity of our singularity. We all have been given karma at birth, the right to our DNA, and our states of being. We have the right to ourselves and what we will become, which is something we forge. The body is matter, and its movement causes energy, we are not our energy, but rather we are our matter. There is no soul, there is no mind, there is the body, which encompasses our journey, and generates the mind. These things must be understood to balance ourselves. We produce wavelengths, these techniques are used to balance our wavelengths, organize our biofields, or control them. The only true form of control is to control ourselves.

Spells:

Passive balance- Self-harmonize the self by using the listening hand technique, to perform a passive balance. Use this technique to listen to other people's balance or to listen to your balance. Understand you are listening to the balance of the bio magnetic wavelengths that your body naturally produces. Organizing your biomagnetism is key to using it. Obstructions in the body can cause displacement of your biomagnetism. The sensory that develops for these techniques allows third-eye usage. Follow the truth and you will find truth.

Tightened balance- Self-harmonize while channeling down your arm. This vibration through your hand will cause your biomagnetism to be closer to your hand. In other words, you may need to move your hands as close as 3 centimeters to balance it. Remember to always move out, back in, and out to get the balance effect.

Focused balance- Self-harmonize while using a pinpoint focus on your palms to strengthen your biomagnetism. When focused you will notice that you may need to move your hands as far as 6 inches from each other to balance, maybe even further depending on your focus.

Advanced: Understand that each technique is for specific parts of biomagnetism massaging. Use a passive balance to find the problems, use a tightened balance to hide and for physical massage. Use the focused balance to guide or manipulate someone's biofield. You can always use these techniques on plants and animals for practice before using people.

Support

These are ways to aid another and to aid your power.

Holy Mancer

Overview: utilizes emotions and emotional bases

Techniques: Emotional control

Knowledge: Divinity

The body has a physical reaction to specific gestures and points of concentration. These points of concentration allow us to measure ourselves to ourselves, as far as our journeys, from our strife, success, and even shortcomings. To become greater is to exercise our divinity, to help with the greater good, and for the right of all. We can create Karama in life, that is why we protect life, for its potential to create more good karma, and its right to do so. To keep even our divinity in check, and our egos, we ask the how and why when becoming divine, even to the point where divinity is more of a societal term. Instead, it is to do good, to be at peace with it, and to help spread good. Measuring your divinity is measuring your serenity, the truth of your actions, and not the outcomes but the source of your intent. Was it for gain or the greater good? Understand sometimes doing good can come with good or bad repercussions, depending on true intent.

Spells: Peace- Trace a line from your eye to above the ear, this line is your peace or divinity line. Place thumbs on your eyes without applying pressure, then place your pointer above the ear, and try to make as straight a line as possible. Take a deep breath and exhale through your mouth. You should feel peace with this line when concentrating on the line connection to your skin, not your hand, the hand is to help make a physical pathway. We are not always aligned with peace, so this may show you if you can achieve peace.

Benevolence- Make your hand straight and place the pinky side of the hand behind your ears, making your hand go up your head vertically. Feel the line you create and take a deep breath and you should feel your benevolence. Again, it may take practicing benevolence to fully utilize this technique.

Righteousness- Take your thumb and pointer and grab your lower ear lobes on each side. If you prefer a line then use the pinky side of your hand below your ears, making a lateral line. Concentrate on your line and take a deep breath. This should unlock your righteousness. Again, exercising righteousness helps this technique.

Advanced: Each technique above is a stance, you can further use these stances with emotion.

Life Mage

Overview: utilizes the body's natural life energy

Techniques: Meditation process, Eternal knowledge

Knowledge: Path of less resistance healing

Our relativity is tethered to our physical bodies. When we have energy problems the source is the body. The body operates in a sequence; all things operate in a sequence, and understanding the sequence allows easier access to the source of the problem. Most problems in the body can have a sequence, especially when dealing with muscular or nerve issues. Finding the path of less resistance is like untangling a knot, pulling on the thread and the rest is easy to unravel. Fix one thing and there surely are more problems, a chain reaction of sorts. Follow the problem to the source, until you find the source. The body is about balance, and redundancy, so when you have a knot, the body compensates for its shortcoming, causing a chain reaction of problems because of a problem. Navigating the problem takes time, and countless situations, eventually it gets easy to follow the problem. These tactics are used in acupuncture, rei Kei, and other healing practices.

Spells: Accessing life energy- hold your hand up in front of you, palm facing outward. Look past your hand and move your hand down about three centimeters. This should allow you access to life energy, or the plasma of an organic house. Do this while in a focused state, you can also use the free flow technique to hone in on the feeling before you try to access the house. Remember everyone is receptive to different houses, and if you do this correctly you may access the green flame. Tighten your hand for a smaller flow.

Living flame- after using Accessing life energy, turn your hand over palm facing up with fingers vertical and raise your hand. This should help you access the living flame, or you.

Spirit sense- the wavelength of matter caused by energetic singularity resonates in the world around us. This perspective can give you a further understanding of the world around you, allowing you to feel the life around you while using Accessing life energy technique. You are feeling energy outside the self not connected to you, existing outside of you, doing this technique in a crowded area or a forest is most effective for practice.

Healing frequency- channeling the brain on both sides of the brain at once, while Accessing life energy allows for further healing frequency, or life frequency which can be used further.

Advanced: the pattern of life energy usually comes as a dark green flame, or yellow depending on how you are tuned in to the natural world. Other colors may represent active systems. Once you tune into life energy you can share the feeling with others. All life is its own, and tune in differently.

Enhancer

Overview: aiding the power of an individual

Techniques: Hidden techniques, Chi charging

Knowledge: bio frequency

We are made of the same materials, with different complexities. We are different as we are the same. We are singularities, which gives us individuality. We are created by our matter, our matter generates our consciousness and our energy, but again in different complexities. What allows us to communicate is our similarities, for example, the nose, ear, eye, and tongue all work the same based on structure, however, can be different in size, color, length, and so on. How we live also shapes us, other than learning, evolution comes from the differences in skill, environment, and food. The more and more we introduce ourselves to new things, the more and more we evolve. We even have differences in sensory variables, meaning not all telecommunication works the same, which may vary from environmental evolution to lineage. Our differences is what gives us flavor, and our flavor varies from the complexity of our DNA.

Spells: Sympathy- We relate to our pain. Can we relate to anything? No, but emotionally we can simulate the emotions of another. To relate to it is to sense it, and naturally makes us better readers both vibrationally, and psychologically. Sensing when someone is emotionally or physically in pain is sensing the differentials between normality and turmoil.

Empath- Sensing someone emotionally is the combination of the skin and the ear. It is like hearing with the skin. We react to people differently, listening to this reaction is listening to them. Feel the body and the skin and focus on your ears to listen to your empathic reaction.

Enhancer- To enhance is to connect with someone at their level, to match or mimic their vibration. You can enhance someone by reciprocating their emotion, either a negative or a positive. You can enhance someone by understanding their state of being, whether it be their fear, charisma, heroicness, righteousness, sadness, depression, or even their love. Sensing them and matching them can help destroy or deploy their current state.

Advanced: You can build power with other wizards if vibrating at the same level by allowing one to gain the vibration allowing the echo effect, to enlarge their vibration levels, creating a connected space. Hiding your presence allows this to take a greater effect on the individual.

Energy

Energy is complex, however it follows some simple rules. All energy comes from some source of matter. You cannot create energy without matter. Our bodies naturally produce several forms of energy, in this section, we will be using these different forces. This will focus on the energy triangle of heat, light, and electricity. Understanding the movement of energy requires an understanding of technology. These are the basic classes of technology: pressure, electrical, temperature, mechanical, combustion, and charge. Our focus is on electrical, charge, and temperature. Electricity is generated by copper and magnets, from the source. There is no negative in electricity, however negative is used to say lack off or another direction. Electricity has a push and pulls to complete the circuit. Once the electricity is used in a load, like a light bulb or motor, the excess is grounded. In some cases, it is harnessed in advanced systems. Electricity is always made by a generator; however, generators must use an outside source of movement to generate electricity. All generators move in a circular motion, constantly exciting the copper. No electrons are moved, if so, this would cause deterioration. The electrons generate photonic energy, and that energy is siphoned through the system. Direct current systems push in one direction. They push through batteries to push a charge. The battery is the charge, which is stored for later, with chemical electrical reactions to hold a charge. Temperature systems use pressure differentials to remove heat, such as fridges and air conditioning units. There is no cold, only lack of heat, heat is removed with these systems. To put heat in you must use either an outside source of heat in a reverse refrigeration system (heat pump), or use a fuel source. Knowing technology allows us to understand systems in the body that can be manipulated or used. Further on this as we go.

Heat

Learn to tap into the body's source of heat, to displace, enhance, or channel. There is no cold only lack of heat or lack of movement. Pressure and heat have a direct relationship, when you increase heat, you increase pressure. Heat has several other properties, like that it rises. The intensity of heat also means the density of heat. For example, how much movement is happening in an area causes heat, the more intense the higher temperature of that area, and as it rises more and more heat is in a cubic inch than there was before, so raising temperature can cause a density of heat. A prime example is a fire, the different colors of fire have different intensifies, and different densities, for example, a blue flame burns hotter than an orange flame, and a blue flame takes up less space than an orange flame. The fuel used is also important, different materials mean different densities and different densities need extreme temperatures to burn. Fire always needs fuel, oxygen, and ignition. Also take note that without the core's extreme temperature differentials and pressure, there would be no atmosphere. The differentials between the earth's core and space are variables needed to understand the creation of an atmosphere. For the gases to stay they need gravity, which has everything to do with planet size which coincides with core size as well. So, to have a core is to reach a threshold of creation to allow the creation of other energies such as gravity. Specific sizes are needed to create a core, and a specific amount of pressure is required to generate heat.

Heat Mage

Overview: manipulates heat to make hotter

Techniques: Sorcery Mechanics

Knowledge: Heat

There is no cold, only lack of heat, which is a lack of movement. Heat naturally rises, and therefore our heat also rises when in extreme differentials of temperature. Understand that when pressure is involved the amount of time it takes to heat things is faster. We are in a pressurized state and use the blood to spread heat throughout our bodies, using a radiant system. A radiant system is a form of heat transfer where a liquid is heated to heat a solid structure, using pipes, where in our bodies the pipes are the veins, transferring heat to the rest of the body through heated blood. We heat our Jing by having our blood warmed by the thyroid and traveling around our bodies to maintain our temperatures. It takes time to heat something, this is the latent property, which can be reduced by our pressure and temperature, so to go further takes practice and patience. To use heat, we must dive into our molecules to heat our bodies since the latent property starts by heating the molecular itself.

Spells: O punch- Channel to the tip of your finger and draw a circle around the other hand. Next, punch through the charge, and feel the difference in heat between your two hands. This should tune you into your heat, the heat around you, and what you can make.

Heat absorb- You need a ring so you can learn to heat absorb. First heat up the ring with a lighter, for no more than 3 seconds. Absorb by pulling on the heat with the rest of the skin, and feel it absorb into the body by pulling away from the source.

Heat focuser- Focus on your palm and intensify your palm by vibrating the palm and pulling in on the skin. Now feel the palm while doing so, and notice the differentials between your palms' heat, and the heat of your fingers. You should feel the difference in temperature between the two.

Threshold squeezer- You should be able to feel the difference in temperature between you and everything else. While in a colder environment, you should be able to sense your temperature versus the cold. You should even sense the degrees of the differential between the two. Not everything is at one set temperature all the time, it may vary, so you should be able to sense the difference and thresholds of temperature giving variable temperatures to your body. All you must do is focus on the feeling of the temperature. Next, take your hands and make a chi ball, about six inches apart. Then squeeze the ball from either side to one inch and feel the temperature variables in the movement. Channel while doing this, then shrink the ball moving in a downward spiral and you should feel the thresholds of temperature.

Advanced: Heat can be used with any distribute technique, as well as weather techniques.

Cold Mage

Overview: manipulates heat to make colder

Technique: Sorcery mechanics, Micro sensory

Knowledge: Cooling

There is no cold, however, there is cooling down, which is like slowing down. To use cold we must disperse, absorb, or redirect the heat. We have a natural cooling system within ourselves by having a pressurized system. We can manipulate the air around us by making differentials in our temperatures, or by moving and dispersing our heat. A cooling system, like a refrigerator, works by removing heat from an area, not making it cold, it removes heat. We will simply be displacing heat.

Spells: Cold channel- Pull your heat towards the center of your body by guiding it along the path of heat naturally created by you. Relax your body while pulling, then tighten to move heat inwards. Do this by channelling the heat from the skin of your extremities to your center.

Cold armor- Use the free flow technique to guide heat inwards creating a current around you, the cold differential around you will increase allowing you to generate a layer of cold.

Siphon heat- Once you perform a cold channel you can pull the heat around you are using the feeling of the heat as a guide, moving it up the body to fill in the heat with heat around you. You absorb by pulling inwards on the heat around you to create a cold space. Pulling heat from parts of the body could create a brain freeze or chills, depending on your point. This is a heat transfer ability, utilizing the pressure of your blood, and the differentials of pressure outside of you.

Advanced: Once you tap into the cold, it is all about where you displace the heat, the cold can be used further with void movement, and earth as well. Layering the self-further can be done, understanding our systems allows for further use, see abstraction.

Fire Sorcerer

Overview: manipulates outside sources of heat

Techniques: Sorcery Mechanics, Channel creation

Knowledge: Fire

Fire is a void in our atmosphere, a space, an extreme in atmospheric conditions. The structure of the material is the base of the fire. The creation of combustion is based on three things, fuel, ignition, and oxygen. Most fuel sources are from organic materials; however, everything can burn given the right temperatures. Ignition is a powerful source of energy that is excited beyond specific thresholds. Remember the anomaly of weather is specifically differentials in thresholds of heat, which allows water and gasses to change states.

Spells: Funnel heat- Using a source of fire, pull the heat using differentials along the self. You don't have to absorb simply guide the heat, pulling up on the arm, on the skin and muscles, you can create a stream for the heat. Understand the thresholds of heat to pull on it.

Controlling base- We can use the mind to control how the fire burns by channeling it to the base of the flame. Connect to the flame by concentrating the signal through your finger. Use a candle to practice. You can make this connection with a clear mind and steady focus. Use anger to focus the mind on the object of ignition and use the focus to control the source of the flame, giving it guidance and direction. You can also pull on the base of the flame and pull up with the fire.

The density of flame- Depending on the temperature, and materials, you can see the density, which is the color of the flame is at. Using thermal imaging, we can see this threshold and see blue fire move as if without itself. You can feel the difference in wavelength with a slow-burning blue fire. You can create this using an Axe spray and a shot glass. Once you see the density you will understand the thresholds of fire, especially in a dark room. Use the threshold squeezer on fire to see its differentials. This can also be used to push on fire, increasing its heat output.

Advanced: Learning to put the mind into the source is the most difficult part of manipulating fire. Focus on the source, and you can manipulate the release of material while the flame is active or absorb the heat to smother the flame. With large flame you can control the space, see space for more.

Light

Learn how to touch the light, and how it moves to understand its power. A braydon comes from the sun, and the sun is spherical, therefore the braydon is in the shape of a sphere, due to its source. Light and the Luxon are not created without a particle atmosphere. If the sun's matter touched the earth, we would have the transmutation of gases, like the aurora borealis, in our atmosphere. So therefore, the braydon from the sun is not the matter of the sun, it is the aura of the sun. Light moves in differently depending on its sources. For example, a fluorescent light bulb has gasses that are in a direct current to create light. Light in a stage light is a two-part system, with a direct current gas bulb, and a second gas chamber to amplify the light. The difference between the two is simply a reflection, refraction, absorption, and stage differentials. Fire and lightning are the purest forms of light on the earth, other than the sun. both produce light, so, therefore, light is just the combination of heat and electricity, in other words, intensity, and pressure, or amperage and voltage.

Arcanist

Overview: uses patterned colored light for various results

Technique: Mindscape building, Sorcery Mechanics

Knowledge: Light

Light comes in 6 primary frequency families, known as red, orange, yellow, green, blue, and purple. Orange, green, and purple are known as transitional colors. When the frequency kicks up, they go from red-orange then yellow, whereas orange is the transition, the same goes with the other two. To harness such energy, one must become attuned to the differences in the feeling of color light. To do this you must pay attention to the frequencies of light in that color. Once you are in tune with different color lights, such as laser lights, you can push on that frequency or replay it with the body.

Spells: Red red orange- Feel the feeling of a red laser light, and push back on that frequency to replay red. Next push the feeling of orange light through the red light by channeling the feeling of orange through the arm while feeling red on the skin. You should feel a rush of heat through the skin.

Pink, purple, pink- Feel the frequency of purple in your arm, then push the feeling of pink on the outside and the inside of your arm. You should generate electromagnetism in a wave as you push out the palm.

Green circle- Create a circle with your arms in front of your chest. Feel the frequency of green light, and circulate the feeling of green, this should give a healing sensation.

Red circle- Create a circle with your arms in front of your chest. Feel the frequency of red light, and circulate the feeling of red, this should give protection or a warding sensation.

purple blue- Feel the frequency of purple in your arm, and push through it with blue, this should give off a magnetic feeling.

Green blue- Feel the frequency of green in your arm, and push through with blue, this should make you feel the magnetic sphere. This has range and scope in the mind.

Advanced: See the color of frequency using the mind as you do these techniques, the more you help the color feeling with the mind the stronger it gets, building a redundancy with the frequency. Using these patterns in light also gives off similar effects. Other patterns also give effects, play around with different patterns to find different effects.

Light Bender

Overview: manipulates light

Technique: Sorcery mechanics, Pathway creation

Knowledge: Sunlight

The intensity and excitement of the sun's matter create an aura, which is called the braydon, the wavelength frequency of the sun which collides with our atmosphere to create light and Luxon. The light is forged by the interactions of the wavelength of the braydon passing through our atmosphere. It requires a particle atmosphere for the light to create a Luxon. The energy passes through the atmosphere as a wave, the crash is light, and the push of the braydon on our particle atmosphere is the Luxon which is pushed downwards on every individual molecule. because of our atmosphere, we get rays of light. because it is energy and not matter, no matter is physically pushed, however, because the wavelength must pass through matter, we get the Luxon, which is the pressure of the energy on matter, meaning the pressure of sunlight on the atmosphere touches us before the light. We call this the Luxon. Atoms that create light have a faster spinning electron surveillance orbit, or the most outer layer of electrons on the atom, which means that the inner rings of electrons are moving just as fast or faster, suggesting the movement level of the electrons stirs up the nuclear frequencies within itself to create the photon. Photons are generated by electrons taking energy from the excited nuclei now vibrating aura. However, it is created, it must pass through matter, by bouncing, reflecting, or being absorbed by matter.

Spells: Light stop- Feel the feeling of light from a light source. The feeling the light gives you when turned on is its feeling. Push on that feeling, and you push on the light.

Light flow- Allow the light to flow on the body, push on it and pass through the light, by pushing on the feeling of light. You can't control light unless you control the source, but you can absorb the feeling of the Luxon on the body.

Light bounce- Using windows, you can make the light bounce through windows by pushing on the light. The braydon is made by any light source.

Advanced: You can push on the feeling of light in multiple different ways, as well as in different shapes and different angles.

Aura Mage

Overview: uses your aura, will see others clearly

Techniques: Third-eye evolution, boundary understanding

Knowledge: Auras

Auras are generated by singularities. Each one includes the 6 frequencies of light. Auras are the way we feel, in this we harness the self and the self's aura, meaning the frequency we feel at the time, which can be manipulated by emotion. Auras can also tell you if someone is confused, clairvoyant, radiant, or muffled by the clarity, or movement emitted by the individual. We are technically in the sun's aura, as well as the earth's aura.

Spells: Aura ball- Make a ball with your hands, and channel you into your hands, should feel your aura in between. Push outwards with channeling, and back to self, all while feeling yourself, you should be able to flex out and in with your ball, by focusing on your aura.

Tuning in the aura- Seeing people's aura change based on their state of mind. Sometimes it can be fuzzy, or clear, and usually has a color the person is exercising.

Frequency of aura- Your aura can be changed by using the brain frequency, Zen pose, and emotional state. Use these to enhance the aura and can learn to play around with an aura ball while in these different states.

Advanced: Don't try to mess with someone else's aura, they must change the state themselves. However, they can be guided to change states. You can learn to play with your aura with distribution.

Electrical

The power of electricity is what has been sought by wizards for centuries. The invention of electricity and the understanding of science gives a greater understanding of the elements, which gives us the truth in magic. This is the era when magic can be explained. Electricity is not a negative, just pressure, or a pull or push in a certain direction. While direct current systems push, alternate current systems pull back and forth. The electrical connection is either there or not, so a switch works to cut out the connection, not necessarily turning on and off, more like connected and not connected. You can learn to pull electricity on currents and light, to the level at which you can pull, meaning to the amount that the body is pulling. Know that electricity will travel to the ground.

Electric Sorcerer

Overview: pulls from a source of electrical power

Technique: Sorcery Mechanics, Cleansing shi

Knowledge: Technology

Technology is naturally organized in a specific pattern to do a specific task. To use electricity, you need to know how things work, for example, understand motherboards are simply connected connections, restricting or amplifying electricity, and storing and dispersing electricity. The source is always different depending on how much is present, which is best known by its wattage, which is the multiplication of amperage and voltage. Knowing the resistance is knowing how much flow you will have, the less resistance the better. Using sources of light as a direct current, we can increase flow using our bio magnetic fields, which is why this technique works on lights so well. Always know what you are pulling. Know how other forms of technology work like TVs radios and such, which are differently shaped and sized magnets and copper to make the electricity move in different ways.

Spells: Electrical pull- Raise your hand, and pull down your hand with muscle and skin, while pulling from light. Have the other hand push down towards the ground, and always do this while on solid ground, to ground. The light naturally establishes a connection between you and the electrical source.

Light brightener- Push on light from a source, and while pulling out with fingers. This should brighten the light. Remember if you feel the light, you have made a connection. The goal is to excite the air in the bulb.

Powering the self - This requires a lamp so that you can grab onto it, and channel through the self, pulling on the electricity. Pull backward on your muscle and skin to pull from a lamp, using the hand that is grabbing it. Channel downwards with the other hand, and this should cleanse your energy-wise. When you do the opposite and push into the lamp or wire, you can make the light brighter.

Advanced: You can draw from outlets and other sources, remember not to touch them directly, or you may shock yourself. Make sure you always use proper grounding, by standing on the ground, barefoot is the best.

Charge Sorcerer

Overview: taking from a source of power

Technique: Sorcery mechanics

Knowledge: batteries

Using a charge is to understand that a battery stores energy for usage and creates energy through a chemical process. The process involves a pin point of metal into a chemical, in which the battery has a push in it initially. This can be manipulated with a proper channel through the battery or can be pulled like needles through the battery. Understand that this requires using a point-of-draw technique.

Spells: Pull charge- Hold a battery device in your hand and pull on the charge, by tightening the muscles in the hand and pulling down the back of your hand. You can even pull a charge from a distance by pulling from your fingertips down your hand. Knowing where the charge is important to pull from a distance.

Drain charge- Feel the energy as you pull from a battery object while making a fist and channeling backward on the arm. Lift to give a pull on the electromagnetism created by the device. You can channel electromagnetism on frequencies through the air.

Channel charge- Pull on a charge and divert the charge with a push, to another or a device, which will do so at the level of biomagnetism you can pull. You will not take in the chemicals due to the physical structure of the device, but you may absorb some of the charge making you charged, you can then push to throw the charge back out.

Advanced: You can do this with multiple devices, and even drain the battery by a percent. To do this more effectively use copper-laced gloves to do so.

Electrical Mage

Overview: creating electricity from the self

Technique: Micro sensory, Pathway creation

Knowledge: The biological and technological relationship

Understand that our bodies are very much like technology. For example, the pump and the reactor can explain the heart and the brain, as well as the heart and liver with the pump and the filter. Our brains, with the flow of blood, cause the creation of our biomagnetism creating a charge through our nervous system to create itself again through the reaction of our skin, giving a redundancy through itself. Our energy system is essentially perpetual, however, requires water and food to rebuild what is used. We are an electrical system within ourselves, and with proper techniques, we can utilize and direct that power.

Spells: AC hand- You are already charged, due to the flow of blood and its reaction with bone and nerve. Make your fingers into a peace sign and touch your other arm. Feel your fingers touch your arm, then feel one finger than the other, then feel the spot without the finger, and the other spot without the other finger. Go back and forth between spots quickly and channel through the arm while feeling spots flicker back and forth. This creates a charge in the arm.

Air static- Take your pointer and feel multiple spots on the tip of your finger. Now do that to all your fingers and pull from the air from all those spots. The more spots you can create the more you can pull from a molecular level. Pulling from a spot in the air creates friction in the air, which cause a charge to be made.

Ground channel- Feel multiple little spots and go back and forth with them to create a charge in your arm. Charge the self then channel, pushing through your arm to push the charge into the ground. Push the channel into the ground while you're charging your biomagnetism.

Advanced: This is a base movement meant for mage use, rather than sorcery. You can match this with other mage works. It good filler for distribution used.

Space-

Understanding the movement of sound is to understand its pathway. When there is no pathway, we call it space. Matter causes the variables in space, and all anomalies are created by matter. Space has its own properties altogether. It is the true emptiness; sound only exists within the thresholds of matter. Truly if not for air, most mystic forms would not work. To be within atmospheric conditions allows life to be possible, and without it, we have space, the blanket of nothingness that separates us from the rest of the universe. Ripples of the universe can be heard within our atmosphere from colliding stars. Though it is a massive vibration, without physical matter the vibration simply does not exist. We explore the second triangle here; sound, vibration and magnetism.

Sound-

Whether it's through our atmosphere, or ourselves, sound holds the key to a hidden reality. Sound is generated by the literal movement, vibrating in a specific pattern, based on the molecular complexity of the matter, allowing itself to be expressed from the singular atom and its reaction with each other. This vibration is carried through air and water. Sound through material is simply based on the density of the solid. The focus is not vibration as much as it is the vibration in which air and water allow the passing of sound through it like it's being played through from the source, rather than it is traveling. It's more like a replay of the vibration through it, and the amplification of its friction, of its physical torture. Sound always requires more than one and cannot travel through nothing. The nature of gases and liquids allows sound to exist, literally gases and liquids' ability to morph into one area is the reason vibration can replay itself in these states of matter, making a sound. No air, no water, no sound, just vibration.

Sound Mage

Overview: channeling sound outside of the body

Technique: boundary understanding, the Meditation process

Knowledge: Sound

If a tree falls, does it make a sound? The movement of a tree falling causes a vibration, therefore a sound would be made if a tree fell. The absorption property of water and air doesn't make a sound. If there is something solid it makes a sound, however air and water together with no outside solid is silent. You hear the air when moving through it, however, that is because you are not just air. Sound can come at different levels, however. Remember it takes two to make sound, therefore an atom other than hydrogen would create a vibration within itself within its movement, this is micro-vibration. Concentrating on this movement will allow you to find yourself, cozied by the micro-vibration around you. Now that you can feel more, then you can feel the whole as sound a multilayered movement, depending on the structure of the vibration. Sound can also be transmitted through electricity, like headphones, meaning we can replay the sound through our nervous system, by allowing the vibration and the connection of the nervous system to replay sound.

Spells: U push- Humming with the "u" sound naturally pushes outside the self. While humming, feel the palm of your hand, sit up straight and align your ears with your shoulders. Concentrating on your ears, hum the "u" sound and know that the that your body makes various connections, concentrate on allowing the vibration to channel down the arms to your open palms.

Song hand- While listening to music, the same thing can be applied, relax the body to allow a better vibration and feel the song vibrate within the body.

Drowning mode- Drowning is when you play loud music, and you drown in the beat of the music. Listen to the second and count all the instruments and vocals playing. Listen to the entirety of the sec of the sound, and continue, as you listen, meditate, and you will notice a portion of the ear will open when you listen to the whole of the song. It is best to listen to multilayered songs for this.

Advanced: These techniques are used to enhance your ability to use sound, and work well with many things, including distribution.

Incanter

Overview: utilizes words of power

Technique: boundary understanding

Knowledge: The language

The structure of the sound is in the current of the vibration, which is the physical pathway for sound to travel. For example, the sound E (ee) is an internal sound. The vibration focuses inward, whereas A (ae) focuses outward, O (oh)is from inward pushing out, and U (you) pushes outward. Other sounds are a direct kinetic language connection, meaning the sound sounds familiar to something in real life. For example, H is represented by heat, and if you prolong the H in ha, you hear mostly a movement of air, naturally pushing like heat. The sound k makes a sound like a spark. Part of this language builds itself into literal words that have meaning based on the meaning of the sound rather than the sound itself. One example is chi. C being air, H being heat, and I being a boundary, literally means what chi is. If you strike a lighter you will hear a ch sound, which is again like chi, which is the chemical reaction of oxygen being taken by the lungs. All these things point to what chi is anyway. Here is a list of sounds that have a meaning in this, which breaks down many of these words in other languages to mean something similar. This is what is found already, if you follow this structure, you can make your own words or learn further from other languages, with other sounds, which some are just a complexity of a sound already, and this structure touches other languages in words they already have, like Japanese, Mandarin, and Sanskrit. Here are some rules for this language. (((E))) and constants in language, the kinetic language is a direct translate.

Spells: Iampoo- Put your hands together and say iampoo, then move your hands apart and back together. You should feel the distance between your hands. You can use this on objects as well. Iampoo directly translates to I boundary, your space a, m matter, p conscious, oo double greater than the self.

Vishnu- With this language, there is an understanding of other forms of existence, which are forms of existence that we don't see, formed by energy and its relativity. Vishnu stands for V grounding, I boundary, sh plasmic, n magnetism, u made outside the self. This may feel like a boundary of the air pushing down on you.

Enahel- Enahel means e the self, n magnetism, a your space, h heat, e the self, l structure. This gives off a powerful feeling of angelicness.

Advanced: This is what is found for a language of the physical literal.

E-ee- inner self, A-ae- space of self, O-oh- outer self, U-you- outside of self, I-i- boundary

K- electricity, H- heat, C- gas, b- nonorganic material, V- grounding, Z- intensity, M- matter solid, Y- organic, L- structure, J- liquid, D- rotation, W- light, Qu- metal, Sh- plasma, N- magnetism, P- consciousness, T- planetary, R- force, G- drop/gravity, V-grounding

Other meanings can be found in other languages. You can listen to the movement of the sound by allowing yourself to channel its flow. building words is up to you and is your choice. This page is left for experimentation.

Conjurer

Overview: empowers the creation of the mind

Technique: Meditation process, Mindscape building

Knowledge: Hearing

The body's matter generates energy. Matter first then movement, then energy. The body's temperature is one of the key elements that create ideal conditions for memory formation and brain activity. The space where you think in your brain is generated by the physical structure, however, is maintained in specific conditions to create consciousness. Our ears work like a microphone diaphragm, creating electromagnetic induction within. The diaphragm picks up the vibration, which is replayed in the brain via electrical signals, creating what we hear. This is very similar to technology, however, generated with flesh. These electrical signals can also be replayed in the thinking space as well. The sound isn't replayed as much as an electrical signal is created and can be replayed with memory. Focusing on certain sounds can strengthen the mind's space.

Spells: Elemental sound- Using the 8 elements, think of the sounds for each element. The sound that is most vibrant in your mind is the element you should focus on. However, that doesn't mean you can't strengthen other sounds.

Movement sound- Now think of the element moving and see it moving in your head, whichever is the strongest is the one you should focus on.

Vibrate sound- Use the brain frequency with the element, which is the strongest within you, now feel the element as well as see and hear it. Then use the sound outside of the self while channeling it down your hand, like a sound signal. The sound may not be there however it is there, don't be afraid to push on the elemental sound. When you get the detail of something it is almost a direct translation of what it is. Work on sound moving outwards away from, you can receive sound, and send it back.

Advanced: Sounds can be used in multiple ways; this technique morphs the sound to you. This technique can be added back to other techniques, to aid or strengthen any elemental-based class.

Void

All share a movement within us, made by the glorious shape of existence. The void has been associated with energy for a long time, however, the emptiness of the void means there is no energy there. However, that means going to space, the true void, when in our atmosphere there is matter, and we are matter. The energy associated with the void is usually by the dark pull inwards, created by wormholes and black spheres. So, we can associate the void with nothingness, and energy storage. To intensify the area within ourselves, and to create a charge, is the most associated energy of the void. The void is associated with nothingness, inward movement, and a downward spiral.

Space Mancer

Overview: uses the power of nothing

Techniques: Sorcery mechanics, Emotional control

Knowledge: Space

True space has no movement, so the vacuum in space only exists because of the thresholds of matter, and the force it creates through its rotation. When we subtract the movement of matter, we get true nothing. So, to know that we travel at 380 meters a second on earth while rotating at 460 meters per second while traveling around the sun which is traveling at 260 km per second in a galaxy spinning at 270 km per second while moving at 210 km per a second, which all these speeds add up to our gravity. Minus all those things, we get nothing, no movement. So, to use nothing is to tune in and ignore our movements movement. To do this you must realize we are in a single spot for fraction of a millisecond. It is more like we are moving through a spot, and we were there, however, there was a movement, so we are never truly stopping but we existed there for a fraction of a millisecond. To feel nothing, you must feel where you will be before your there, so we know we are moving even when we are not moving physically. This is used for tuning in with the greater universe.

Spells: Movement of nothing- Clear the mind and feel neutral, with no emotion while standing. Walk forward and feel yourself drag behind you, understanding that we are constantly moving and never in the same space. So to move while moving is redundant and strengthens your movement.

Using nothing- While in a neutral state, feel the grasp of your instinct, and flow with it. While using nothing, the body will manifest its movement, to follow this listen to your core, and flow with what wishes to go first.

Space ball- Put your hands in a ball form, while doing this pull away from the ball using your skin and muscle. You are creating a space that should give the space some flow. While using nothing, form a space ball for best results. Remember nothing is minus everything including you, so to feel nothing is to not feel the self. When creating a space ball, naturally other movements will fill the movement of the emptiness.

Advanced: Once you learn to harness the power of neutrality, you can fill the space with other movements, such as heat and electromagnetism, and other things as well.

Void Mage

Overview: pulls in from the magnetic sphere

Technique: Sorcery mechanics, Qi connections

Knowledge: Singularity

Physical nothing is space, this is the physical literal. Imaginary numbers are called this because they do not exist, like negative numbers. Therefore everything, not nothing is positive. While all matter is positive, most of it is neutral. Things that create a singularity usually are super positive matter. For example, life is an energetic positive, while planets with cores are super positive, and stars and black spheres are considered ultra-positive. biology naturally creates itself into singularities, all the way down to microorganisms. Our DNA gives the body the code for singularity, which is us anyways. We can manipulate that energy by creating further heat density within ourselves, or a greater charge within ourselves.

Spells: Pull inwards- Tighten your muscles and pull to the core of your body. The magnetic sphere contrasts with you as you pull inwards towards the self, allowing the energy of the magnetic sphere to pull through you.

Singularity charge- Let your hands drag through the air, then tighten your arms and pull your arms inward as well as your core. As you do this you should feel energy absorbed along the body.

Void palm- Raise your hand and push against the energy of the earth. Push outwards while meditating. Feel the effect it has upon the air and the energy around you. Pay attention to the differentials of energy around you. Now do this while pulling inwards. You should feel an emptiness and a buff to your singularity.

Advanced: These techniques are utilized best by using this as a stance. Using stances can aid in charging with other movements.

Spiral Mage

Overview: the power of the inward spiral

Technique: Micro sensory, Pathway creation

Knowledge: The spiral

The 192 polygonal star naturally has a spiral in its make. The spiral is created by the structure of the multiples of 192. This star naturally creates a 3d illusion of the spiral and a sphere within a magnetic sphere, otherwise, it would appear flat outside of relativity. The shape naturally separates color, and sound with its thresholds. The importance of the spiral is within the complexity of higher atomic numbered elements, as the outward spirals create a movement for the inward to move and so on through the structure creating the spiral. The image can be used to understand and feel the movement of the spiral. This will allow for quick memory learning, by feeling the movement. This works best when light or energy is applied to the structure.

Spells: Spiral beam cannon- Create a brain frequency and twist it in the brain. Push inwards from the opposite side to create a twist. Put your hand in a "V" shape around your third eye, charge, and point. Use the signal hand technique to further this spell.

Spiral absorb- Draw a spiral on yourself with your finger. Feel every point your finger touched and pull in on that pattern. It should naturally pull in energy to that center point.

spiral punch- Charge your finger and draw a spiral with it in front of your fist. Then punch through it, you should feel the charge of the finger when doing this.

Advanced: It is easy to use this with other movements, such as heat, light, and electricity. You can make the spirals push out as well, by reversing the pattern you create. Eventually, you can make spirals along the body without your finger, allowing yourself to charge the body quickly. This also pairs well with distribute classes.

Advanced

This is in-depth on power created by our relativity, to further understand reality. The advanced movement of auras, explosions, and lightning allows for a further understanding of spatial reality. Tesla Towers put out an aura of electricity. The sun and anything that create a singularity cause an aura. We cause an aura; in essence it is like we are creating light within ourselves. The light of the sun is not the matter, but the aura, we know this because the matter of the sun when it hits the earth creates the reaction of the Arora borealis. So, the braydon the sun produces is an aura. Combustion is an expansion from a point, a chemical reaction that violently pushes outwards quickly, or an implosion which is a condensing of energy in a spot quickly. Lightning is like a crack in the sky, created by pressure, and differentials of temperature. These are three advanced understandings of spatial reality.

Abstraction Mage

Overview: focuses on the outside of self in omicron variation

Technique: Sorcery mechanics, Qi connections

Knowledge: Abstraction

This focuses on the boundary between yourself and the outside world around you. Our bio magnetic spheres push out against the magnetic sphere but are still encapsulated inside the earth's magnetic sphere. These are two systems at once, and there is a natural barrier between you and the earth. Know that your biomagnetism, your heat, the kinetic flow of blood, and the grounding of your bones, all go into the creation of your singularity, which is all these variables together, making simultaneous movements creating your reality. The separation between our complexity, and another creates several layers of reaction.

One layer of reaction is like touching outside of our barrier, making a connection via our focused biomagnetism, to allow a pathway from your physical to your barrier and its barrier's edge, meaning it has a paper-like existence, a transparent barrier that is not there however produce by the self. This is our aura within an aura. If you can see these variables and the number of variables that go into understanding variables, with tools you can learn to minus and add variables into the variable understanding. With the understanding of technology, we also start to understand more about our existence, and how simple reality truly is. This is a form of abstract understanding. The key is knowing one barrier is created by another, from the multilayered structure of the skin to the blood moving throughout the body, creating layers of movement even with one not moving however existing and affected by the subtle heat differentials between skin and blood. We also have a bone and nervous system which creates variables as well as multiple reactions within each other. Meaning the variables of combination, if you must go deeper, have a limit limited by what exists.

Spells: Crush- Feel the edge of the self and your biosphere, or light body, and feel the spot outside of you, and make it smaller. You can also open and close your hand while focusing on a target.

Expansion- Feel the edge again, then point at the focused spot with all your fingers from one hand, and then expand them.

Pull upon- Feel your edge again and pull the edge towards you. Use hand motion to gain a full connection.

Advanced: This is a stance. To focus more use Sith to build up focus on a spot. This also pairs with a dark magic very well.

Combustion Mancer

Overview: focuses on implosions and explosions

Techniques: Sorcery Mechanics

Knowledge: Combustion

Combustion is always caused by three things: fuel, oxygen, and ignition. These are the key ingredients in combustion. The focus however will not be on these ingredients as much as on the actual movement. Remember, combustion requires fuel, a source of matter to ignite. These techniques do not require you to blow up anything, however, allow the movement of combustion in your biomagnetism.

Spells: Pinpoint focus- Channel down the arm to your fingers pointing at an object, while the hand has every finger aiming at a spot (including the thumb). Feel the focus generated between your fingers and push through the center, using the channel.

Focus and pull- Focus on a spot using the star hand (previous position) and pull on the spot.

Explosion- Focus on a spot and point and channel down through the star hand, and open hand to cause outward movement or movement of explosion/expansion.

Implosion- Focus on a spot and use an open star hand. Close to causing implosion movement, while channeling backward on arm.

Advanced: Utilizes this focus with heat to increase potential, as well as pairing with Sith to increase focus.

This is just the movement of heat, and can be paired with Abstraction techniques as well.

Lightning Sorcerer

Overview: focuses on harnessing the power of lightning

Techniques: Sorcery mechanics

Knowledge: Lightning

For true lightning, you need proper conditions, which would be a contrast in temperature/pressure, like a low and high front colliding. The differentials between cold air and warm earth usually cause lightning. Regardless, this is like combustion, you will learn its movements to allow for static creation. Static uses friction, these techniques use air friction to create static.

Spells: Clash- Channel down the arm with muscle while pulling up the arm with skin to create a clash.

Air drag- Focus on a point in the air. Reach in then out of the molecular, zoom in then out, and pull on the air after you weaved some focus in the molecular level. Then pull your skin towards the body to pull the focus to you. You are dipping into the molecular, yet your molecular focus is large than that space, it is beyond what you can see, however, you are seeing it, so focus should be achieved this way.

Call of lightning- Use air drag up in the air and pull towards the ground. You should be naturally creating pressure to call upon lightning.

Static bolt- Use clash on both arms and air drag with both arms at the same time in a chi ball in front of you. Push outwards with lightning.

Advanced: Use with Arcanist and the purple, pink, purple spell. This should aid in it. Conjurer always goes with lightning, and Incanter has words to intensify the movement of lightning, depending on how strong you want to go. You can put energy in the molecular, and gain back the same amount of energy coming back, but strengthened due to energizing the molecular itself. Use the visuals of lightning to conjure lighting with this spell class.

Scaled-

This is the aspect of the bigger picture. We must understand our place in the universe to understand further our purpose in the greater ecosystem. Our viewpoint must take a large view of the greater whole. What is offered in the scale can be invaluable, as well as powerful. Here we tune in our senses to a new level, while extending power to even change global aspects. While this is rare, learning control and understanding pathways can allow for a greater purpose, and sometimes we are called to make a large change. Responsibility is key in using these spells.

Celestial

Learn your place among the stars, your purpose on this planet, with the aid of father sun. We are all part of a physical and spiritual ecosystem, what we are we give in death, and we are worthy of what we have done in life. That is the only thing any one of us is worthy of is our actions. We are written under the stars, gazed upon by the sun, and nurtured by our planet. What is written is only up to interpretation, the key to the interpretation is personal, and no one will truly understand your fortune as you do. Remember things like luck are all written in number patterns determined by time and existence and come to us in threes. These patterns are within understanding nigh omniscience. Nigh omniscience allows us to read patterns by making a system that is varied and vague, we fill in the details of our own life using this series of patterns.

Sun Sorcerer

Overview: pulls from the sunlight

Technique: Third eye evolution, Sorcery mechanics

Knowledge: The sun

Earth is constantly in the ray of the sun; its rays reach us from the sun to earth within 8 in a half minutes. It takes 15 to 18 hours for the sun's matter to reach us, via the Aurora borealis. The sun rotates about once every 4 weeks. We are following the sun in space. Knowing the details of the sun allows us to use these details in meditation.

Spells: Sun pull- Using a pull channel technique, connect to the light of the sun, understand its glory and connect with what the sun has given you. Focusing on a molecular level, feel the sun pull over you. Feel its warmth flood across your body.

Third eye absorption- Use a pull channel technique while in a meditative position, and pull the sun from your third eye in, pulling downwards on your stomach muscles. Open your inner mind to the sun's chi and attune yourself to the feeling of the sun. Pull on your inner mind and allow a charge to flow in. and feel your reaction to the sun.

Sun blast- Harness the feeling of the sun into your hands in a chi ball. Pump the chi ball, which means to flex, then relax, flex, then relax, flex, then relax. That's one pump session, then push the heat and the energy from the sun outwards. Focusing on the feeling of the sun and moving that feeling is one way to use the energy the sun gives you.

Sun breathing- Electricity can flow on light. Pull the light of the sun into your mouth, by breathing in the light. Knowing that electrical signals can flow on light is enough to pull the light and Luxon into the body. This will charge your systems, and you will feel the feeling of the sun pump through your veins. If you do this right, you should be able to taste the light of the sun. This should allow you to taste the differences in light within an area in any condition regardless of the sun.

Advanced: This is a situational usage, to use the sun more look at memory mancer to harness the sun even when not in the sun. Feel the feeling of the sun even when not in the sun just through memory.

Star Mage

Overview: knowing your place among the stars

Techniques: Meditation process, Sorcery Mechanics

Knowledge: Reading stars

The stars that give the most meaning, are the stars in the sky lined above you during birth. Some internet sights can give you the stars in the sky based on your birthday and place of birth. When interrupting the stars, understand it always has to do with you and your interpretation. During interpretation, you should know some of these rules on reading: association with the sign, similarity, or familiarity to the sign, deeper meaning of the sign, confliction of signs, differentials, positive and negatives of sign, student of, and general representation of the sign. This is good for self-knowledge interpretation.

Spells: Place in the cosmos- Understand your place, not on earth, but in the stars. The truth of you in the greater cosmos, in the universal ecosystem. Surrender to your serenity in the view of the cosmos and meditate on your serenity.

Nirvana- Meditate on your chi, your elemental type. Whatever you are in the universe it is what you are the deepest inside of you. So, the answer for nirvana is simply inside of you. Use the eye lid focus technique while meditating on nirvana, and know your cosmic place in the universe, which is revealed to and is based on you and what you are. There are layers to chi, so nirvana is about four layers outside of you. Nirvana is like your home in the cosmos.

birthrights- The stars that shine over you in the place you were born are your birth stars. Use the knowledge to interpret your stars.

Advanced: These are skills for self-knowledge. No one else needs to know your place, only you.

Astral Mancer

Overview: become a beacon on earth within the cosmos

Technique: Qi connections, Sorcery mechanics

Knowledge: Nigh omniscience

Nigh omniscience is knowledge based on patterns. 0-9 16 and 18 give patterns used for organization. These are analytical tools used to separate multiple forms of information. The secret is knowing what to use, and how to use it. For example, sometimes it's the aspects of the 8, with a ⅔ ⅓ pattern, like 7 with a family. Can also be like nine and 5, sharing properties of abstraction. The use of nigh omniscience is best in science and not in situational knowledge. It can be used to predict with other tools, such as the possibility to probability, to the truth. The possibility is any form of the situation, the probability is fact giving greater detail to the situation, and the truth is when there is nothing left but what happened or happening. History and creativity like to be in 3's, knowledge likes to separate in 4's, and processes always come in 8. These are techniques used when creating further tools.

Spells: Earth drag- while in a neutral state, meditate and feel the drag of the earth through the cosmos. Feel the gravity and the magnetism of the earth, is like feeling the outer free flow technique, it just redundancy what is already there, which makes it stronger just knowing about it. The sensory of it is innate, so focusing on it makes our innate senses stronger.

Earth tuning- This requires you to be part of the greater ecosystem, minus the societal system we make. What is your place in the greater ecosystem? There is the basic ecosystem, then there's the greater which includes everybody. What are you to other people? A guide, a protector, a healer, and so forth. Do you only exist for everyone else? We are made for companionship so technically we are for the people, but the ecosystem is greater than what humanity has seen so far. It is deeper, it is natural.

Contrasts- Understand the difference between you and earth, the contrast in materials that create two different relativities. If you acknowledge your singularity, the singularity of the earth will acknowledge you, giving yourself redundancy. Meditate while feeling contrasts with the earth. Remember the difference are innate.

Advanced: Find your place in the universe. We are bred in a system that when we give redundancy to what is already there, we strengthen it. What did your parents do? What did your grandparents do? If you work on what you were bred to do, then you will strengthen a primary purpose. If you haven't been exposed to everything, then you may never find your meaning.

Earth

Utilize the power of the earth itself. There is more earth than water, the deepest part of the ocean is predicted to be 7 miles, and the earth's crust is predicted to be from 43 to 60 miles deep. There is more earth than water, it's just not seen. Regardless, even the water meets the earth. These styles focus on vibration, the magnetic sphere's charge, and gravity.

Vibration Bender

Overview: uses the sense of vibration

Technique: Meditation process, boundary Understanding

Knowledge: Vibration

Vibration travels in a direct root of structure and considers the density and redundancy of that density. Multiple levels of vibration can be achieved, building a redundancy of vibration, and allowing for intensity. Knowing the structure of items, and areas allow us to have a greater impact. Most structures follow a mathematical structure from both an atomic standpoint and a multilayered standpoint. You can have vibration within an atom, but like sound requires two for the vibration to travel. The secret is 864. Most things stand on a 4 for applied pressure, however, can increase with gravity giving it a 6 on impact, but if the structures are vibrating, it gives the push more of an 8. 864 can also give a representation of pressure, the higher the pressure the more closed in the angle.

Spells: Vibration all connect- Nothing is ever still, if you put your hands on something and listen to the object move on a molecular level, you'll notice the feeling never stops, and when you go deeper you can feel it vibrating. When you are inside you can sense the smallness of the area, compared to the sky ceiling outside. This is because of pressure differentials. Tune into that feeling.

Channeling vibration- Vibrate your hands by channeling just your hands. You can push this vibration through higher vibrations adding to it. This includes the air or the earth. It also allows you to push through objects, to send your vibration through the micro-vibration that already exists. Start with layers of vibration, from the atoms singularity, to the molecules singularity, to the structures singularity, then the singularity vibration from the earth, air, to the vibration of the fabric of reality, and the vibration of yourself. You can listen to all of these at once, it is innate.

Vibration sense- You can use multiple senses to feel a vibration, both your skin, and ears. You can sense vibration in a space, or sound in a space with your skin. You can sense pressure in a space as well as with your skin.

Advanced: Pairing this with mindscape ability will allow you to further your vibration sense. This pairs well with the following styles: geomancer, tree mage, alchemist, and flood.

Geomancer

Overview: utilizes the magnet sphere through the earth

Technique: boundary understanding, Qi connections

Knowledge: The magnetic sphere

The center of the earth is about 1,600 miles deep, and the magnetic sphere itself reaches up to 40,400 miles. This requires massive amounts of energy to continually produce this, which is mostly an aura produced by the core. Regardless of the thickness of the earth, magnetism pushes through. The geothermal energy from the earth warms us via the magnetic sphere and does so less at the poles. This energy radiates within or rather pulled by the structure of the core. The ground of the earth holds energy, a charge of 30 nanoteslas can be found in most of the earth at the equator, where the poles can be up to 60 nanoteslas. The goal is to feel the charge of the magnetic sphere in the earth. It was here before us and we are unaware of it due to it being normal, however, it is there. Tuning into the magnetic sphere is like tuning into the world around you.

Spells: Raising earth- Create a connection with the earth, feeling its charge, and its nanoteslas. Once you feel the charge pull up on the nanoteslas. You'll find you can pull on a larger area once you connect. You can stomp your foot on the feeling and then lift on it as the vibration floods. You can also lift your hands through the air and feel the charge the earth gives the air.

Push through- Once you lift a field of nanoteslas, push through the feeling of the earth using the feeling of the earth to push on, (push means to channel through) pushing through the lifted field, using the all-connect feeling as you make yourself one with the earth.

Lowering earth- Reverse the feeling of lift by pulling down through the earth, using the earth as a fulcrum.

Geosphere- Understanding that the earth creates a shield using its poles allows us to see the sphere that we create through our poles. Feel your poles, head and feet, while standing in a horse stance, concentrate on the poles of the body.

Advanced: This is a stance, that can be used with others to maneuver other movements, generate other movements, or stack with other movements.

Gravity Sorcerer

Overview: pulls on gravity

Technique: Sorcery mechanics, boundary Understanding

Knowledge: Gravity

Gravity pulls at about 32 ft/s2. This is the rate of fall on earth. You can tune into gravity with various movements due to the vestibular systems, which maintain postural equilibrium in the inner ear. It is important to understand that structure has a direct literal correlation with how it applies to the physical. Why recreate something that already works? The body has many systems that detect electrical frequencies in various forms or patterns. We can sense pressure as well when tuned into an area. We are accustomed to specific environments that we forget the sensation of the differential, like the difference between being outside vs inside. There is a cubic difference inside vs outside, that creates different pressures due to the differential alone.

Spells: Gravity fall- Lift your arms straight at shoulder level, then dead drop them and catch them at chest level. You will feel a pool of energy, this is gravity you are catching. This is how you access the feeling of gravity.

Totem usage- Find a dense object and use this as a fulcrum to pull gravity through. Use the feeling of gravity to pull through the object to affect an area or thing.

Fulcrum- Using the gravity of your relativity, pull through the earth and then through the fulcrum. Gravity pull- Pull from gravity after tuning into the force of the earth.

Advanced: You can make a good spot around the totem, or even use the spiral technique to bunch up the gravity. You can pair this with many things, especially space abilities.

Weather

Learn to bend the air, or move through water, while making it rain. The differential in the temperature of the water is basically what makes the weather. In other words, the condition of the cloud makes the weather. Without clouds, it would just be differentials in air, following patterns of heat rising, and cold falling through heat, again only difference in the air is temperature.

Air Bender

Overview: manipulates air with heat

Technique: Sorcery Mechanics, Micro Sensory

Knowledge: Air

It is known that heat rises, we also know that extreme differentials cause heat transfer, and we are at a constant at 98 degrees. To take heat we would have to be in the presence of chemicals that cause heat absorption immediately, however, glycol is not rained. So therefore, our heat transitions are more of an absorption process rather than a dispersion. We must physically make the dispersion by pushing out and can aid the absorption by pulling in. being at 98 degrees means we have a constant variable, whereas the rest of the environment may not be at that variable, which we are in, therefore our touch can transfer heat due to our differentials in temperature. When the weather is hotter, we can absorb heat and displace it into other areas, this technique also works on hot objects, or fire, to displace the place of burn. We can create pathways to displace heat as well as move heat in the air as well, creating streams of air to cool with the air. These only works because of our heat differentials.

Spells: Arm flow- Create a path on the arm with pinpoint technique, feeling the entire path, and make it spiral around your arm. Then pull on the heat differentials to pull the air across your arm.

Hurricane ball- Tighten your pinky then relax, then your ring finger relaxes, and do this to every finger then your palm then starts over at the pinky. Next, tighten your inner hand and then circle the vibration around your hand, do this with both hands. Now feel the heat differentials and pull on that to create a ball of air. The center should be calm if you have it done right.

Heat reach- Extend your arm and tighten your fingers, and push out on heat, pull back your arm while in a tightened formation to move the air with your hand.

Advanced: There are various ways to manipulate wind, with electrical directions, and with any of the distribute classes, especially Pathway maker.

Water Bender

Overview: gaining control in water

Technique: Sorcery Mechanics, boundary understanding

Knowledge: Water

Light only travels ¾ the speed in the water, however, sound travels 3 times faster in water. The light of water only travels less due to its density of physical structure, compared to air, however again due to its density sound, caused by vibration, travels 3 times faster, however, is direct in its path due to water pressure and temperature. The colder and the more pressure directs sound downward, whereas in cold air sound travels further, and in hot air, sound travels faster. In water, the sound is more intense than in the air. This goes with vibration as well. The temperature in water causes heat to be more direct, flowing with heat, or around it. The connection we make within ourselves is enough to direct water, especially when in the water.

Spells: Water flow- While swimming, feel the current flow past you, as you sense the water flowing past your entire body, you are making an electrical connection for the water to flow on. Concentrate on the flow while swimming to allow water to flow past you.

Vibration push- Channel while in the water and push past your body, feel the vibration flow beyond you. You can push further with the all-connect.

bubble cling- Make your body static by using the clash in water, use this on your core. As you create biostatic you will notice bubbles cling to the body. Play around with this at different levels of depth.

Advanced: You can use various techniques underwater. In this specific space, you may be able to pull off a lot more than while on land.

Rain Sorcerer

Overview: manipulates the sky

Techniques: Sorcery Mechanics, Cleansing shi

Knowledge: Weather

Tuning into the weather is like tuning into another world. The weather is effect by land geological terrain and presence, however, that is only at the surface. Weather is another world within a world, it moves with and without the earth creating worlds of movement. While weather is on earth it is in its sphere of existence, which we call the atmosphere. You are either part of the earth watching the weather move, or you are one with its movement. Understanding your perspective is either redirecting or directing. We are in ourselves a diaphragm, and we can move with the weather or be our relativity. If you are affected by high and low pressures, you are one with the atmosphere, best way to go about this is to be in the spot in which the weather can be aided. You cause a redundancy, empowering the weather. You redirect its power. The direct is one with the earth watching the weather move, they create weather, using its land structures as tools for the weather.

Spells: Low spot- To affect anything you need line of sight. You can pull down on the atmosphere from underneath by using the gravity pull technique.

High spot- by pushing up on gravity you naturally create a high spot. Another way to do this is to generate pressure with your hand and push the pressure upwards. To generate pressure, tighten the hand and pull inwards on the skin, while pushing out with the arm. Connect with the spot using abstraction abilities, outside of your line-of-sight bubble.

Cloud pulls- Use the low spot technique underneath a cloud to pull rain down. When you build high or lower pressures you can direct where the clouds may go, then use what fills in that space.

Advanced: be careful when you do this to avoid lightning crashes unless that was your goal. Remember knowing the weather and its direction, and knowing the terrain as well helps with weather direction. When a spot is under high pressure it is in a clam. A calm is usually the best place to exercise weather abilities. All these techniques are much stronger the higher you are, so doing this on a mountain top is optimal.

Mind

Dreams can reveal time, strategy, and warnings, recognizing a dream is vital to navigating the dream. Dreams can give feelings that can be used to recognize situations. The mind gives us physical pathways that can be navigated or tuned into. Learning to tune in is key when using the mind. Learn the layers of the mind, as well as use greater mind techniques, which is the key to psychic ability.

Dreamer-

Learn to control your dreams, understand them, or even navigate the dream realm. The first rule of dreaming is understanding the purpose of sleep, which is to rejuvenate the body. Remember you don't always have to dream, sometimes it's best to get that rem cycle going, which is active in dreaming but works best when we are unaware, the deep sleep. Deep sleep is always within the self, dreaming is always in the self. Your dream self is always a reflection of the self, and in walking is the state of your whole, the DNA you are. Sometimes dreams are used to solve issues you have in the physical, things that psychologically cause turmoil can find you in sleep. Wrestle with these dreams to find the interpretation that will solve the issue. Some issues are harder than others. Sometimes the dream gives you nightmares and sometimes could mean what is coming, or what to expect. If you haven't faced your fears, fear can be another reason for nightmares, regardless something could be reaching out to you. Remember that all things dream, so sometimes we must interact with other beings or creatures in our dream, for they dream too but at a different frequency and within themselves, as we are within ourselves as well.

Time Mage

Overview: learning to sense time fluxes, and the truth

Techniques: Sorcery mechanics, Dream law

Knowledge: Time

Time is a constant, regardless of if it's an illusion, it is a constant. It may not be tangible, but that does not mean it does not exist, for that which is in time exists, or did, and that which doesn't exist in time does not exist. Time flows, and creates moments, and moments can be better revealed with details. Time dreams are always in a specific way, they are always first person, always related to the self, 3 weeks ahead of time, or longer, but are more constant at and real at 3 weeks. These dreams usually last from 10 to 30 seconds. Deja 'Vu is usually something that has been seen in a dream as if you saw it. The feeling of Deja Vu is the first moment of capturing a time of passing or seeing the future. Once you see a moment it will be easier to identify DeJa'Vu.

Spells: Phasing in time- Throw a punch and feel one second. Now throw a punch and feel the milliseconds. To do this feel every action of the punch, in sections. For example, when you throw a punch, several other mechanics are happening, focus on those mechanics. This is how you exercise your feeling of time by sensing every second and every movement of that time. One second is a constant, but how much you can fit in one second is variable.

Deja vu- Once you have a Deja Vu, sensing a Deja Vu is like second nature. It is like a truth that is happening now that you have already seen. So, to further your ability, when you see a Deja Vu say something that will awaken you to the time, like "I've seen this before". At this point, you are now making your own timeline, not what has been seen. You can break out of the normal and change time itself just by changing your reaction with time. This is how you become a butterfly being, a being with no specific fate. Rule your fate.

Frequency changers- Change the frequency of an area and you change its time. because of the rotation of the earth, friction and electricity is created at a gigantic scale. The charge that is, is the charge the earth creates. It is grounded by the consistency of the earth. The earth's relativity is its ground, so when we use time, we use electricity. Change the electrical frequency of an area to protect it through out time.

Advanced: You can change the area with different frequencies, specifically the frequencies of eternal knowledge. You can use phasing time with martial arts to increase your movement speed. Deja Vu is a gift from the sun, use them well, or change your fate. Deja Vu feelings are associated with feeling the truth.

Mind Soother

Overview: studies various forms of communication

Techniques: Hidden techniques, Unlocking the innate mind

Knowledge: The mind

To access the mind is the same way we access it ourselves. For example, if someone looks left they are looking into truth, right is imagination. To understand someone, you have to know these 6 things. Right is imagination, Left is truth. The upper mind is visual, the middle mind is sounds, and the lower mind is kinesthetic. The eyes are considered the center of the mind. While listening, which we can listen with multiple systems, the acquiring of information in multiple systems, allow the reaction to happen, so to listen is to listen to their listening. Remember sometimes you won't get a result, due to being no problems in the person, this works better for those that need help.

Spells: Listening hand- Using the back side of the hand, relax and listen. Feel the listen, listen with your skin. This is just another form of listening. You can listen, see, and feel with other parts of the body, connected by the brain. Open the full of the brain opens extra sensory. To do this requires exercising extra sensory like what is given.

Making responses- Use the ear and feel the connection and listen to the truth of the target, by placing the hand on the left side of them. You can feel responses that they need to hear, or want to hear, by connecting the ear with your skin, knowing the connection between the two is your skin. Feel the vibration the target is trying to hear.

Influencer- You cannot control another, but you can influence what they want or need by listening. Some commands you can give, are feelings to which they respond. For example, using gentle on animals allows the approach to the given animal. Make your hand feel gentle, by focusing on that feeling in the skin. You can use various emotions, such as sternness, comfort, caution, and even fear.

Various minds- Animals tend to think different to us not just because of their place in the ecosystem, but because of their variables in sensory. Dogs tend to communicate through the frontal lobe, while cats are better at projecting. Whales and dolphins communicate with various senses, at a larger scale then us. Birds tend to respond to sounds better than us. All things communicate, however, they communicate at a different levels, so the results you may get when psychically communicating may vary.

Advanced: Various mind techniques pair with this, such as genjutsu, emomancer, and mirror mancer.

Dream Walker

Overview: Learning to explore the spiritual plane

Techniques: Meditation process, Dream law

Knowledge: Planes of the dream

The complexity of us goes on multiple levels, understanding how to walk you need to access your subconscious and gain control. After you have established control of yourself in the dream then you can walk the many planes of life, which are like you, on multiple levels. For example, the plane of fire is like the core of the earth, and electricity is the vibration in the earth, and the earth's core. These all make up the physical plane. There are more planes, however, the only one you need to know is the physical. The advanced section will have a place you can visit in the dream.

Spells: Full body sleep- This is simply listening to the body while going to sleep. To do this you must practice relaxing the body with meditation. Once you have done this a couple of times and you can relax on command, then you should be able to fall into sleep while fully relaxed. This is full-body sleep.

Leaving the body- When you leave your body, you must be in a meditative state, and may only be able to do this after enlightenment. There is no other reason to project yourself into the dream, other than exploration and understanding. To project the inner self is to leave the body out of the back of the mind. You will see your body in harmony, meaning what your body wants to be not what it is. Remember it is a projection of yourself. You have full control of your projection by accessing certain parts of the brain. You will always be the controller, not the control.

Dream control- When you wake up from a dream, meditate to go back to bed with how you would change the dream, allowing you to access that part of your mind.

Advanced: There are several places to go. There is the wastelands, a desert plane of dunes, where only a few can travel. There is the healing temple, with the gardens of the giraffe elephant hybrid, who walk amongst the reeds. Remember the water is much deeper than it seems. There is the elder council, the circle of tree seats that the old gods used for those who traveled. Every planet has its own. Then there's the fairy realm, not welcome to humans, but a sight to see if you're invited. There is the subconscious of the forest, remember your reaction is your own, the forest reacts with all of us differently. It is no one, but everyone's. There is also the dream shack on a pier in the middle of Alaska like terrain, with secrets to fighting that which can also dream and is not human. There is the hall of devils, where those who seek to be one wait. Then there's the dwarven spaceship, ripped apart and full of mysteries and treasure. be careful what you choose, for some secrets are meant to be discovered on their own.

Psychic

Learn to harness the power, or to manipulate from a distance, even to see from different angles. This book does not include the ability to move objects, but how to move the mind in different aspects, and enhance the body as well. These techniques are advanced, however, simply done with practice.

Mirror Mancer

Overview: seeing from multiple perspectives at once

Techniques: Mindscape building, boundary understanding

Knowledge: becoming a machine

Dimensions are created by the physical, from stars to planets and even people. People are singularities, in the fact they create a dimension within themselves, our perspectives and point of view, because we matter, and have that innate property about us. We are created by our physical with set values, what makes us different in our experiences. We are machines, once you start pressing your own body's buttons, you are in control of the machine that you are. Once you gain the fact that your carving of yourself is by honing your machine, you are ready to understand that there is one existence, one reality dictated by the physical. However, we can and have been able to access the mirror realm, which reflects your reality, which can be created by the mind using the mindscape technique and physical mirrors as aids.

Spells: Viewpoints- Choose a place and gain a full view in your mind of the place, use the mindscape technique of seeing around you. Now choose a position and make a viewpoint if your basic position. Now remember that viewpoint, make another viewpoint upside down, above you, below you, to the left and right of you, and at different angles. Now throw a punch at those angles and view those angles in your mind and strike from every angle at once from your center. Should be able to see from all those angles at once and strike as one.

Reflection- Put yourself in a mirror chamber where you get a reflection that goes infinite. This will help you with visuals of yourself from different points of view. After getting a view do some movements and see those movements. Then use the visual in your mind space and strike with infinite versions of yourself all at once.

Mirror traps- The mirror trap is the same as a mirror chamber, which works well on negative entities and demons. It splits their reality trapping them in infinity. This is great for manifestations.

Advanced: This goes well with other psychic styles, and does well with genjutsu, and mind soother. Use the reflections to perform soothing hands from multiple points at once. Add energy to your movement as well to enhance this.

Projector

Overview: creates channels for the inner mind pathway

Technique: Mindscape building, Pathway creation

Knowledge: Projecting

For this you will need to have a strong mindscape of the self, projecting is combo sensory based. Understanding your sensory retainment, or variable of sensory is important. These techniques require the use of touch. This is not astral projecting, but rather physical projecting. However, the order in which you project may be different based on bloodline sequencing. Just know you are projecting your senses.

Spells: Voice throw- To project the voice you need to protect the throat and visualize the fullness of the throat and its actions. Vibrate the throat and mirror the self elsewhere, you can also create a tunnel for the sound to follow displacing it elsewhere. Also, you can use the portal mancer next to utilize the voice.

Mind punch- This requires you to move the brain frequency out of the mind. Make a pathway of the frequency with the mind outside of the body. Then power your vibration through the pathway you have created. This requires lots of practice with brain vibration. Once you unlock the vibration in the brain it should be easier to create it even without using channeling. You can make a mirror image vibrate or vibrate your mirror image to also use mind punch.

Projecting self - You can project the self with abstraction or sound. Tap into using the sounds e and u, which pushes you into the u. With mindscape, you can create an image of yourself doing something around your vicinity to also project. Using the feeling of iampoo also allows projection, as well as utilizing your ear touch senses. The best way to project is using the eye-touch combo. Focus on the skin and your eyes at the same time to unlock this.

Imaginary Parkour guy- Imagining a being that runs beside you while driving is the best step to creating a projection. Imagining outside the body is one way to create a projection, adding vibration to your projection, or adding color wavelengths, sound or movement is one way to create a projection. Making multiple projections and making them move in different ways is another technique to strengthening your projection. You can use your imagination with this, so you can imagine Godzilla, or characters from your favorite show, large beings, small beings, monsters, heroes, and so forth.

Advanced: You can add any movement with this to enhance and can use other extra senses to do this as well.

Portal Mancer

Overview: focuses on abstract connections

Technique: Mindscape building, Cleansing shi

Knowledge: Portals

Understanding portals is understanding the void. Via heat, you must create a point of entry, at the same level of frequency as the point of exit. Remember you won't be able to make a physical portal, but you will be able to project the mind and body, the energy. Like projects, this is a form of projecting and moving your senses.

Spells: Create portal- Pull down on heat and squeeze the thresholds, then expand, do this in two sports and push through while they are on a specific plane in time. So do the movements while holding a specific time, each holding the same time.

Double arm portal- Put your hand fist to fist, after generating a portal, then thrust both in over each other. This is the first movement to start doing this. Next, strike through the portal with one and the other and feel the result of the other, you should feel heat and movement.

S portal- Project a tunnel in an S movement. This connection is good to move energy through. It is also very good to use projecting sound. Remember to create the path using your brain frequency.

Shadow clone- Making one is as simple as pretending to see something, like making an image run next to the car while driving, pretending something is jumping from pole to pole, then adding variables such as depth, frequency, color, texture, energy and other variables such as contrast and density you can home in making it visible. You can also use this technique to do this for portals, visually seeing it or making it up creates a redundancy that strengthens what's there.

Advanced: Work on mindscape with this and add movements to this as well.

Layers

There are layers to our existence. From the mind negative that creates a field around us, to the body's natural wavelengths created naturally by other systems. These are layers of the mind-body.

Shadow Mancer

Overview: uses the lack of light

Technique: Third-eye evolution

Knowledge: Shadow

First, there is no shadow, only a lack of light. Obstruction in the pathway of the light is what shadow is. In the mind, if you used eyelid focus training, you would discover there is color in the mind, surrounded by darkness, or lack thereof light, what the mind naturally creates. This focuses on the creation of light through our matter, now we can't make light, but we can use tools to provide light, so that we may use the reflection of light within our eyes. The residue of light within the eye allows for the use of it. For these techniques, we will be using the physical pathway of the eye.

Spells: Summoning shadow- Face a light and stare at it to create a blind spot in your eyes, this should only take a minute. Once you have a blind spot, focus on the spot, focus your eyes specifically on the spot, then pull your focus back out, then into the spot again. This gives it depth, then focus on the spot and detach yourself from the spot by breaking away from the focus hold. If you do this right you should be able to make a spot in the air the color of the blind spot. Use a piece of paper to make the spot float and absorb on the paper, allowing you to show people the shadow of your blind spot.

Shadow burst- Summon shadow and then put your hands around the shadow spot, feel the shadow, and amplify that feeling with your hands. Tighten your hand and push outwards with your ball to realize it, with one hand under the spot and the other behind it and push on the feeling of the spot.

Call upon shadow- Remember the feeling of the spot. Now manifest that feeling by recalling the feeling of the spot with your hands. As you learn to manifest you can summon the shadow without using the light. You may have to do this several times to recall the feeling.

Advanced: This is a filler and a direct way to affect the spiritual. Use the body to echo the feeling of the spot.

Shade

Overview: traversing the physical literal spiritual

Technique: Mindscape building, Cleansing shi

Knowledge: Dimensions

There are many planes of existence, in other words, multiple layers of energy are created by the physical plane. To gain entrance to the outside plane around you is to break the barriers of the natural body. Our brain and skull create a field around us, holding our negative mind (the residue of thought and senses creates a negative, like in photos). While it's not truly negative, it is referred to as this, an absorption property of the brain, absorbing the reflection of light, in specific frequencies. This is the negative. The barrier the skull and the brain make is like a geosphere, holding it within itself, creating a barrier based on our physical structure, what makes us a singularity, and separates us from the spiritual realm, or the plane of earth, the outside world. The best way to understand this is to understand the 4th and 5th dimensions, density, and contrast. The density of us varies and differs, and the contrasting feeling always us sense these differentials, like the differences between us and everything else. Once you are aware of the contrasts, then comes how to condense yourself and revert your senses to the outside world.

Spells: Entrance- Use the cleaning shi technique of moving into the spirit while you have your mindscape active. You should be able to feel outside of your barrier by doing this. You can also shrink your mind barrier by concentrating on the center of yourself.

Manipulating EU- Understand that the outside of your light body is the outside of the mind field. It moves with your body, so to manipulate it all you must do is move your body.

Opening- Use a doorway to create an opening to walk through by creating a threshold with your mind. Since a door is a threshold all you must do is hold your light body at a door using the mindscape sight, of eye touch combo. Compress your energy by pulling inwards then walk through the door and feel the threshold move over you. Use the doorway as an entrance into the spiritual and perform entrance at the door to move through.

Shade walk- This is like making a tunnel. While walking through the opening technique, leave your vibration behind you, making a tunnel of vibration of where you just were. Being aware of the self is one way to let the self-go. Feel the self and let go of it while moving forward, leave your presence behind and blend into the environment.

Advanced: To understand what's on the other side, visit Residence. There you will have a greater understanding of what awaits you on the other side.

Naturalist

Overview: become one with your actual wavelengths

Techniques: Sorcery mechanics, Qi connections

Knowledge: The body produces an electromagnetic field, from the blood pumping and the reaction within the brain, which then is giving power to the heart. So if the heart is beating the brain is functioning. The heart pumps all our lives, creating these fields of heat and bio electromagnetism. Tuning into these fields is simple, knowing how they look, not just by how they feel, is a little more difficult. For those interested in using a thermal imaging camera and or a line camera, both of which can give you an idea of your fields. The camera is only one portion, feeling the biomagnetism is quite simple, in fact where you put your concentration can help cause redundancy in your biomagnetism, making it stronger.

Spells: Field wavelengths- Your heat thresholds and electrical thresholds are caused by the movement in the body. Use the free flow technique then focus on the body feeling of the free flow, strengthening the power of the free flow technique, making it echo with the redundancy of focus.

Focusing wavelengths- Once you focus on your field, next hold out your hand and focus on the feeling of your hand. This will cause further redundancy strengthening your field. Focus on every detail of your hand, even down to your palm lines. You'll notice an echo if you have multiple layers of redundancy.

Shaping wavelengths- Push on your palm lines to accelerate energy outwards. The naturalist focuses on what the body is already producing. Focus on spots around the body, with every detail, every cell to create further redundancy. Focus on shapes or movements of the body, such as a heart beating, for your field to flow on, and feel the flow of your field.

Advanced: Naturalist mix well with distribute styles.

Dark Magic-

As naturally as it is abused, it is within you. To evade enemies, to use their minds and bodies against them, or to even unlock the beast within you. To understand death, bloodlust, and even mimicry is the concept of the predator. This is not to give you dark power, as much as it is to control dark power with the law. Tame the dark side, then there is no dark, nor is it just light, now its reality, both dark and light, like how a shadow is made. Learn to control the beast, activate it or hide the beast, or understand the purpose of blood magic. Knowledge is like a shackle to the dark, without it, it's just superstition and fear. Let us be in control of our inner beast.

Stealth-

Learn to hide your presence, in several different ways. You won't be able to go invisible, however, you will learn to displace, minimize or change your presence, which can be enough to throw off foes.

Stalker

Overview: Hides their vibration

Technique: Micro sensory, Hidden techniques

Knowledge: Concealment

Concentrating on where you feel is very important. These skills use these focus techniques to displace their presence, to hide their life presence, our constant vibration. One way to do this is to focus on the area you are touching. Go barefoot and feel only your feet and the contact it makes, think about only the contact, feel only the contact, and you will be in the contact. Now go on your hips to the ground and feel the surface area of the floor. be aware of your surroundings, indoors is hard than outdoors, because of your you-to-area ratio. It's easier to hide your presence in the open world. What materials are near you can change your presence in hiding. Use biomagnetism concentration on multiple parts of the body. Remember these techniques, because to achieve inanimate presence, which is a lack of life energy, you will need to use both breath concentration, and channeling to hide presence.

Spells: Air hides- Put yourself into a neutral base. Jump and feel the drag of the air. Now jump again and release while jumping, this will naturally drag your presence in the air. The more focused you are on your body the more you will drag your presence in the air making your vibration dissipate into the air. Let it flow around you like a bat in the sky, making your presence dissipate further. You can add this with minimize to eliminate your presence.

Ground hide- Lay down on the ground and feel the connection between you and the ground. The more you concentrate on the connection, the more your presence is in the ground. Feel the fullness of your body contact on the ground to disperse your presence into the ground. You can also push your presence into the ground using channeling.

Water hide- Take a neutral stance while in water. Use the cross-stream technique and create a chi ball in the water. Keep your center of balance while allowing the water to direct you where to go. become one with the water. While doing this, swim into the water with full contact of the mind on your body. Allow the water to flow around you and hide you in the water. To do this further, use your mindscape ability while in the water and see your surroundings, utilize the ear-touch and eye-touch connection to be one with the water.

Advanced: This mix very well with minimizing techniques in the following style tracker.

Tracker

Overview: minimizes presence to sense the presence

Technique: Hidden techniques, Meditative process

Knowledge: Flavor

Jing is our flesh, which holds our DNA. The platelets in our blood do not hold our DNA. Our Jing holds our DNA in every cell. We are a solution of signal, our signal being our DNA at the cellular level. Those who are more selfish give off a stronger vibe of themselves, while the selfless are harder to detect. It's easier to find evil this way, they give off a strong flavor of themselves. You can minimize your flavor potency by exercising well or using the following techniques.

Spells: Minimize- Pull from your extremities to your center. Concentrate on feeling your core only. This will minimize your presence.

Sensory immersion- Take the minimized stance and center of the self. As you listen, listen with the ultimate feeling technique, which is hearing, seeing, and smelling with the skin, while using your mind's eye.

Feeling presence- Next, you are going to use a redundancy on your senses to listen. Use the ultimate feeling technique then concentrate on the nose eye and ear, then use the skin to encompass all. This doubles your sensory field. Use this while minimizing the scope of the area.

Advanced: This stance works well with stalker, as well as with instinct mage. You can use any earth skill to further listening to presence, hiding presences, and sensory immersion.

Mimic

Overview: makes their presence feel like something else

Technique: Hidden techniques, Unlocking the innate mind

Knowledge: Mimicry

Learning to feel like an object, is to blend in your presence with an object. This skill can be used to help blend in, limiting your presence, however, does not mean you are invisible. It is all about detailed senses. You can discern that things are fundamentally different by their structure from the molecular level to what we see taste and hear. Using sense together is the key to blending in. Sound and sight are always using a disguise, but to feel is different. Using taste and feeling we can discern the differences between materials not by the texture but by flavor. The flavor of an object is how it feels, and not how it feels. In other words, the molecular pattern of the atom is how something feels, and how the atom structures itself with a bunch of atoms is how it tastes, the difference is in multilayered structures. So, the energy of the atom vs the texture. Singular structure vs multilayered structures are the difference between how we taste through feeling or what we are feeling.

Spells: Inner mimic- Taste the feeling of an atom, sense the touch of its multilayered system. Use the inner mind to discern the difference but give the similarity of the object. Using trees as mimic is first. Feel every valley in the tree's bark, the dirt tangling with the roots, and even the leaves with water in them, that differential brings a specific feeling. Now feel the whole of the tree and use that feeling within your mind. Going any further on animate objects is considered the dark side, so to ignore this, we acknowledge that you are your matter, you have a specific feeling so use this with hiding your presence first.

Outer mimic- Everything has a frequency that bounces out at light level as what it is. The idea is to give off a frequency that mimics another at that level using the feeling of the item. Mimicking something means you give off the complete structural sense of something, due to the knowledge of taste touch, like the tongue knowing how everything tastes. The tongue is simply an extension of touch, having extra sensitivity to heat, and is protected by the mouth, because of its incredible in-depth texture sensing, as well as its infinity to taste due to structural design. In other words, the tongue does serval other jobs as well as touch.

Shifting- Shifting from one feeling to another is like going from a glass cup to a ceramic cup, or from tree type to plant type. It is easier to change with something similar in touch.

Advanced: Coming out of mimicry is like using presence hide. Use stalker style to cleanse out of mimicry. As well as shifting to a neutral base.

Body

The body has multiple systems we can use to our advantage. The difference between every system is the uniqueness of our bodies.

Bone Mage

Overview: channels deep infusing power with the bone

Technique: Qi connections, Hidden techniques

Knowledge: bone

Bones are porous within their structure. bones hold a charge within their structure, allowing the bone to be felt. There are multiple ways to feel your bone. The nerves ground to and charge the bone, creating redundancy to feel the bone, as well as aiding in a process known as hematopoiesis, the process of making blood cells. The bone can hold a charge, that is why we can feel our bones, and feel the pain of breaking them. The skin has a layer known as subducti, which separates the skin from all other tissues. The skin has its own system, separating it from the bones' systems, creating another redundant layer of energy. We call this the skin and bone spell, the realization that your skin does not touch your bone. Meaning the skin grounds to itself not the bone, and the bone grounds the nervous system. All have a different reaction; this feeling allows access to skin and bone. This focus is on the feeling of the bone. We can draw power from its structure and hold power within.

Spells: bone draw- Feel the skin and bone realization, the pull from your bone with your skin outwards. bone fill- Push inwards on the skin to the bone, you can use this to fill the bone with frequencies or energy.

Bone gun- Channel through the core of the arm, pushing through the bone and releasing outwards in the palm. Advanced: Using bone fill with multiple frequency types or energy movements, to unleash or save for later.

Skin Mage

Overview: uses the skin to amplify abilities

Technique: Eternal knowledge, Qi connections

Knowledge: Skin

The Skin has the innate property of absorbing energy, like the ability to absorb sunlight. These properties can be utilized in different ways. They can also be amplified by the skin. This property is found in crystals, that when present with magnets amplify the properties of the crystal. Using our blood's biomagnetism, we can amplify our skin, as well as absorb the biomagnetism. We can use things like light, heat or electricity, even gravity, magnetic sphere, feelings, emotion, vibration, and other things stored in the skin, or we can use it as a passive magnifier, mostly amp what's there, and use it as a tool rather than specializing it. If you have chosen a path, however, it can be a powerful specialized tool. To start this both, we have to listen to the skin in the skin and bones spell.

Spells: Amplify- Know that your skin can amplify energy. When pushing outwards on the skin, allow the skin to amplify it naturally. Concentrate on your biomagnetism in your skin, by causing a redundancy of concentration, then push outwards again and notice the refining of the energy output, giving the energy from the skin more texture and density. Pushing out on your forearms works best with this.

Absorb- Pull inwards on the skin, to absorb the energy around you. If you use the skin and bone spell, you will further the amount that can be pulled in or pushed out by including jing.

Protect- Use your mind-eye technique with the skin and bone technique. Feel the whole of your skin and know the more you feel the more redundant your system is, adding strength to it. You should feel your biomass become more refined.

Advanced: With these techniques, you can absorb even more energy into the body. This is great with energy techniques.

Blood Mage

Overview: the force and the flow of blood

Techniques: Meditation process, Cleansing shi

Knowledge: blood

The secret to blood magic is understanding types. blood cells don't have DNA within them, instead, they have antigens, a, and b, both, or none. Your blood type flows best with you, using your type works best. When making a spiritual weapon, blood can be used as an ingredient or amplifier, it is best to get it drawn professionally. Infused in a handle would be the best way, however, using blood outside of the body is not usually necessary for blood magic. In reality, blood magic is flowing with the blood in your veins, using the push and pull of the heart. Focusing on your heartbeat and blood flow is the first step to using blood magic.

Spells: blood charge- Concentrate on the heart, and feel it pump. Put your hand on an artery, like on the neck, to feel the flow of blood. Pull in between pumps. Time the heart and pulse with it.

Focus blood- Time with the heart to push out, or to pull in. Push out on the arteries and pull in on the veins when your heart beats.

Blood flow- blood is greatest when in the body, move with your blood, time the heart, and move with your blood, like moving with your chi, however this time flow with the blood. The dance of blood is when you can move with your blood and move with your body, to channel outwards on a beat during the movement or cycle inwards to pull in.

Advanced: blood can also create a charge, so using this with energy types is good, as well as using gold to cleanse the plasmic space of blood. blood can also be used for enchanting, please draw professorially, there is no reason for spilling blood.

Old magic

These are the parts of the body that are naturally taken advantage of by others. Mastering these allows you to be able to counter dark magics or old magics. We call them old because of the misuse of these abilities in the past. Now to control the old ways with new understanding.

Fearmancer

Overview: learn to control the power of fear

Techniques: Emotional control, Micro sensory

Knowledge: Reality of fear

To use fear, one must conquer it first. Fear is truly only present when it is present. Paranoia is a manifestation of fear and not the moment. Fear of retribution is a motivator for work, however, is not true fear. Fear is when the kidneys activate, and the adrenaline starts to kick in. That is true fear. While it is common to fear animals, they are only a threat when they are there. Fear of human intelligence and the capabilities of humans is also when they are there, however, sometimes the greatest fear is that intelligence allows for an unknown factor, and this is what we call fate. To beat fear, one must simply not be afraid or anticipate the fear beforehand to prep for a situation. It is good to expose the self to fear to truly understand the self, and your reflexes, to help tune in proper reactions to fear, or to test the fight of flight and to control that experience. Remember it is ok to live, a flight is ok in certain situations, learn to fight for another day, is one thing, though when in a party, react with flight unity. Don't abuse the power of fear either, just because you can doesn't mean you should, however, what is dangerous about these techniques is physically using them on another. To test this use yourself first.

Spells: Reveal fear- Start by focusing on the listening hand. Target the side of the body below the waist. Use a listening hand to pull on fear, by tapping into your fear to create fear. Fear is a stimulant and a chemical, but will affect the target in multiple ways, such as flight or fight.

Replay fear- Once you gain control of fear, you can replay the reaction of fear over and over. Remember you can have control when in fear. Gaining control of fear means being in fear to use fear. You can activate this by putting the self in a protective stance, do or die stance. Fear that you can be defeated, and now you are afraid. Use that fear to control the fear.

Quelling fear- Let go of fear by meditating and breathing out of your mouth. Feel the fear release. You are now in control of your fear.

Advanced: To truly be a master of fear means fighting fear in meditation, by seeing your greatest fear, and understanding the reality of that fear within the actual physical situation. Use the deep meditation technique and focus on your fear, when you get the answer you will get your true fear from the medium. Let go of the fear, and fall into deeper meditation once you have let go of the fear. This is one way to algin the chakras.

Necromancer

Overview: understanding death and utilizing its tragedy

Techniques: Meditation, Cleansing shi

Knowledge: Death

The universe is coded, and this code is to know what happens after death. The truth of death is the lack there of life. In life, we have our matter to produce our consciences however this luxury is not for the dead. Death has no word; it is simply silence. In most cases, death is a release of energy. If reincarnation exists, it is passive, it works without us wanting it, so now in death you become nothing, giving into this allows the passive way that has worked forever. Even reincarnation in families can exist, usually towards your cousin or related family, not your spouse's family which means never in your own kid's family. It can also work as organ donors, that we could reincarnate with a match type, meaning we match ourselves, which allows us to be various beings if reincarnation exists. Literal death is the most scientific. All we know is we only live once. Ghosts most likely are recordings of frequencies of the last moments of life. Ghosts cannot think, and most ghosts exist ignoring the law. This is the way exorcisms are possible. The power of death is to avoid it, truly it is the power of life. The mitochondria gain power through their structure and reaction to matter. The power is always within, with a passive 3 being the micro chromosomes in you mitochondria, the intermembrane space is 6, and the outer membrane a 9. The 9 is insulated, holding the power within the mitochondria. These batteries hold lots of power within them. The secret is to harness the power of mitochondria for the self. Although it is powerful, it uses a battery.

Spells: Vengeful spirit- This is a passive-aggressive stance. Destroy an enemy with the spirits they have killed. Even the greatest of heroes that have slayed someone has to face the life that they took. Without respect for life, they become a target of revenge. Every life has potential, so taking away that potential is a great sin. All can be redeemed though. Redemption is for the greatest of us and the lowest.

Release of death- The realm of death is accessed through three levels of wavelengths. Nothing should be in death, however for some reason something insists on living in death, which makes the existence of beings possible however illegal and against nature. Nothing resides in nothing and only nothing. because of the existence of malpractices, Dhaka exists.

Hand of living death- Pull downwards at the cellular level. To do this you need to understand the mitochondria. Focus on the battery of the cell and pull inwards to ignite its power. Focus molecularly on your hand to access the power of the cell. You live, so this is the recycling of energy that you're feeling, or consuming. Feel this energy then use it as you will as it moves into the rest of the body.

Advanced: White necromancy should be the focus, to preserve life. Use this to preserve life.

Instinct Mage

Overview: harness the power of instinct

Technique: Unlocking the innate mind

Knowledge: You can code your instinct, that is the glory of being human. You can do this with martial arts. There is a mental aspect as well, like cravings, that can be trained via knowledge. For example, orange juice can help with the withdrawal of cigarettes. This is because vitamin c helps the immune system, so you can train your body to crave orange juice when you think you have an immunity issue. When you use the full of the brain, there is a take-back, always feel the cooldown of an exercise after unlocking ferocity. This may require relaxing the body via meditation or jogging off the excess adrenaline. Unlocking the brain is not information, it is sensory, and movement. To get super smart you need information. Using the rest of the brain is using the body, so when unlocking our instinct, we unlock the body as well.

Spells: Double instinct- Push out twice on your instinct to create a double instinct. This projection of your instinct can decrease reaction time. This will engage your cat-like reflexes.

First instinct- Push out using the feeling of red. Red is the bases for defense and the bases of instinct. It can also come with anger. To fully be in the red, unlock the innate mind while pushing out on red. Focus that power and anger on a task, like working out. Control the instinct in red.

Internal instinct- Meditate and concentrate on the gut. Feel your body's instinct and move with this instinct. While tuning into your internal instinct, use martial arts to train your instinct into what reaction or style you want to use.

Advanced: These are powerful stances and can be used as a base for fighting. Practice further by using instinct in situational circumstances.

Distribute

These are ways to deliver energy. The same ways can do more than others, some use other aspects to create ways to move energy, and others are sheer raw power in technical movements. They can all add feeling, or energy to the specific movement, as well as be aided by technology. These movements are advanced stages of wizardry, to arm yourself with ways to deliver your new knowledge of the elements.

Versatile-

This is to utilize hand mastery in channeling energy. It can be done in various ways, there are some simple ways to do it.

Triangle Mage

Overview: using various hand techniques to push and draw energy

Techniques: Pathway creation, Hidden techniques

Knowledge: Superstition of essence

Understand that we react with the elements and push the elements as they are. We create auras, which are made by us but are not us. Essence is essentially our body heat and biomagnetism. We can't leave our essence on things due to singularity laws. However, we can push energy, not pushing matter just movement, once you understand that we just move heat, and electricity around then you understand the pathway techniques.

Spells: Single hand- Create a looking glass with a single hand. Tighten your hand completely to where the second knuckle on each finger is bent. Look between the thumb and those fingers. Push horizontally with your hand while looking through it.

Tri poses- Create a triangle with both hands, thumbs, and pointers touching to create a triangle. Now create a field by channeling through thumbs and pointers. Look through the field and push through it with your eyes. You can also push forward with thumbs and pointers and then look through to create a field with your viewpoint.

Heart pose- Make a triangle again and turn it into the self. Then channel into your thumbs and pointer to create a field that goes with the heart. This is a natural healing pose for the heart.

Advanced: This can be used with Laser mancer, and with other movements.

Gunner

Overview: pinpoint blasting

Techniques: Pathway creation, Micro sensory

Knowledge: blaster

The body is all connected and works in unison with itself. These techniques are different ways of pushing energy, which requires an understanding of the 6 energies we can manipulate. These techniques are techniques for almost any aspect of this book. These skills can be added with other skills to fill when using. This version of the distribution is based on pinpoint channeling.

Spells: Gun blast- Curl in your pinky with your ring finger while pointing with your pointer and middle finger with your thumb up. You are making a gun with your hand. Concentrate on your fingers and channel through your fingertips.

Open Palm blast- Using pinpoint sensory, feel the wrist and forearm, circle around the wrist and forearm to charge up, then channel through your hand.

Charge up- Pull back on the muscles in your hand, then push through while tensing. This while charge and cause build up in the hand.

Advanced: Movements go great here, as well as other martial techniques. Don't be afraid to create different moves with these three basic forms.

Swordsman

Overview: uses slashes through energy and with it

Techniques: Pathway creation, Micro sensory

Knowledge: Sharpness

These techniques require honing down on the channel, to create sharpness. They require you to make an edge within your fingertips, to allow energy to move in a narrow line. They work well with hands and can be added with technology and tools later.

Spells: Slice- Make your hand straight, channel out through the tip of the pointer or your fingertips, then move your hand through the air, this is a slice.

Cut- Make your hand straight, and channel pull back on your pinky or your fingertips, and then move your hand through the air. This is a cut.

Refiguring- Slice through a cut or cut through a slice to counter or display. A cut should open a gap, that the slice can utilize to project further. Hone in a cut with a combo slice/cut.

Advanced: This is used well with movement. Moving the arm in two motions, cut on the way down, then slice on the way up. Also you can add sharpness by focusing on the very tip of you fingers in the tightest it can go, you can also use your fingernails to add sharpness.

Utilitarian

These are energy ways of delivery, a system within a system. They are techniques specifically for specific energies, however, can be used with others if done right.

Weapon Mancer

Overview: creates light weapons that can be filled

Technique: Sorcery mechanics

Knowledge: Shaping

These techniques require light and heat. Pulling the heat within your hand, then pushing it on the light in a certain shape allows it to form. There is always some light, so this can be used in the dark, however, works better in light. Using a thermal imaging camera, you can practice creating and holding these shapes of light. However, it is not necessary to perform these skills.

Spells: Shield stance- Push out on your forearm using a light stop technique to form a shield. Use the mind's eye to develop the shield form.

Bow stance- Make your hand into the Vulcan peace sign and close your fingers. Push out on outer fingers with a light stop and use the other hand to connect to it. You should push on either side of your hands the light to create a bow. Again, you can use the mind's eye to visualize the bow. You can make the arrow into any movement you want.

Weapon maker- Put hands into ball form. Push the heat from either side through each other. This will create a vacuum. In this space, you can fill with mind thoughts to create something of your choice. Usually best to fill the space with a feeling or movement. Shape the light into the shape of a weapon and feel with feeling and light to make a weapon. Can add technique to bow and shield stance.

Advanced: All of this can be added with movement, as well as feelings.

Signal Mage

Overview: creates signals to care wavelengths

Technique: Micro sensory, boundary understanding

Knowledge: Antennas

These techniques require an understanding of antennas. One way is to feel the palm in two spots, channel back and forth, then push down the arm, with the hand in a V shape. This will allow the usage of the antenna effect, which allows you to channel sound, light, and other movements through the wavelength you create. This will amplify your power if you do it right. This is a multiple energy move and works with several other skills.

Spells: Sound channel- Create a v hand, then pinpoint the palm from one side to another to create a channel and push down both sets of fingers. While doing this you can channel sound to your hand and feel the sound move through your fingers as you create a frequency.

Light channel- Create a v hand again, and create a channel, push on the feeling of light while doing this to feel the light travel through your fingers to your target.

Cricket blast- Pull inwards on your hand and excite the cells, tapping into the mitochondria at the cellular level. Channel through your hand while doing intense v-hand, to create a bubble-like push. This causes an amplified pulse wave.

Advanced: Add movements and sharpness, or intensity to make a stronger v hand. You can channel the zee sound to create more intensity.

Ray Sorcerer

Overview: pulls and distributes energy at the same time

Technique: Pathway creation, Micro sensory

Knowledge: Preparation

These techniques require multiple movements at once to achieve. They require both dark and light chi, one as a push, and one as a pull. Daoist's philosophy speaks of the different chis as hard and soft, black and white. When using these techniques, we will be calling upon both chis together. If you are not a strong chi user, you can use the physical pathways given below to build a pathway that eventually will move easier when you apply chi.

Spells: Charge beam- Push through the center of your arm and pull back on the skin to create a beam.

Destroyer mode- Channel up on your legs and channel out on your palms, this works well when palms are facing down at the floor.

Charge cannon- Put both hands together, and push through the palms, while pulling up on your arm's skin.

Advanced: In one direction or another if you use your mind's eye you can see the chi movement, the black, and white. You can add movements to it, especially light or electricity. You can also add this with the Kaioken to give a push, or add raw intensity as well. Use the pull technique of the move to pull energy from around you to add some power. This style works well with technology.

Power

With technique and knowledge, learn to unleash energy at larger levels.

Laser Mage

Overview: focuses on tight pathways

Techniques: Pathway creation

Knowledge: Creating the weapon

You can choose what to do with your body. If you understand that the body is a machine including the brain then you can use yourself as such. We are given set values to achieve body harmony, the experience is your voyage throughout life. The brain is used for accumulating information which is essentially your life. The choice is to use the brain as a tool, or not. This next section focuses on brain frequency techniques.

Spells: Eye blast- Activate your brain frequency, push the frequency through your eyes, and release past your eyes.

Brain laser- Spiral the brain frequency left to right and channel through the brain through the center brow, basically out your third eye.

The dragon breathes- Channel brain frequency through your teeth. Connect your teeth by opening and closing your jaw, almost closed, you want to touch your teeth then open and close with teeth never touching them again. Push through using air to carry frequency once you made the teeth connection. Connect space with vibration from the upper jaw and lower jaw. Push through using the upper and lower jaw and add breadth to carry a frequency.

Advanced: Teeth are like bone; you can enchant them with frequencies. Again, this is a major application, if you do not want to then don't. However, the side effects seem to be positive. Always use proper grounding.

Path Forger

Overview: focuses on creating large pathways

Technique: Pathway creation, Mindscape building

Knowledge: Mind's eye setup

Choose your moment, by using the mind's eye technique, and by understanding your area and surroundings. To truly affect an area, it is always best to start with an area with little movement. Advanced training requires using the mind's eye technique with movement and maintaining the focus on the body and sensory on the area. This requires two states of mind to due, so maintain the eye feel of the body, with the mind's eye technique, then without anticipation follow the change your body is flowing through. You can gain an acute sense of the area, using the contrast of objects. Gain this focus and continue with the spells below.

Spells: Hand cannon ao- Using your "e" with the brain frequency technique as a source, push on the "o" with "a", making a path in "o" and making "o" follow the path on your arm. In other words, if you push on "a" it should echo to "o". If you can push on your "o", which is the space around you, then do that to push through. Use your arm to push through "a/o" to gain greater effect.

O large path- Visualize behind you then push an image of the location through you as if making a pathway in a large area. Use the full of space and create a pathway redundancy for air to follow. Resemble as o with the mind's eye, create a body as a channel, push from back to the front of the body and feel the difference in space, a, and o.

Creating space- Use a path that you see and channel with brain frequency, to fill the e and use e to fill a and o, so in other words, use your e to push outwards to create a space you now control.

Advanced: This goes well with weather usage. Remember to visualize the space you can see, and feel the whole body while visualizing the area.

Pulse Mage

Overview: utilizing the molecular to the seen pushes and connections

Technique: Eternal knowledge, Pathway creation

Knowledge: Visual pulses

To truly see a pulse you must see a pulse in reality. Trees grow simultaneously within themselves, growing at every angle at once, and only changing to their environment, seeking the path of less resistance. They grow at once with themselves, this is like a physical pulse, only in slow motion. When you attempt a pulse, you will need to reach the cellular boundaries, and push along that path, through every cell together and at once.

Spells: Force flood- Channel through your arm while focused on a molecular level in your hand. Channel through the earth in a flood with your hand. If your channel is through the molecular you should be able to do this.

Force push- Channel from every cell outward, pushing from the cell not through. Push as a tissue first to get to the cellular level if having trouble. Remember you are the cellular of yourself. Push from every cell outward, push from and around the cells altogether, like pushing from multiple parts at once.

Reverse flood- Channel pull back simultaneously from the area you already push into. That makes it easier. This technique goes well with absorption techniques.

Advanced: You can use this with multiple techniques.

Martial Arts-

These skills add a style of fighting to martial styles that already exist. They incorporate different aspects of the game. Beserker deals with incorporating energy with your strikes, with prefight techniques, like charging up for battle. Chi blocking gives several styles of strike tactics, used for stunning the opponent. Genjetsu attacks the fighter's focus, distracting or redirecting attention. Each style is unique, however, do not incorporate every aspect of martial arts. There are ways to add to the physical arts.

Beserker-

These forms concentrate on channeling and honing energy. There are three styles, upwards channel, outwards channel, and inwards channel. These are stream, thunder, and pressure styles.

Stream Style

Overview: uses upward streams to enhance blasting

Technique: biofield manipulation, pathway creation

Knowledge: Micro flexing

The Human body has a charge to it. When we create pathways, we are pushing through our energy field. To create pathways, you simply must flex in a repeated order within a specific area, which can eventually, through practice, cause you to micro flex. If you have something causing blockage to your pathways, you may find this a little more difficult, or may even pass out. Remember you are not causing physical pressure; you are causing a current to flow off you. Micro flexing is flexing a group of tissue within a family, like flexing a piece of the muscle, not the whole thing. This is almost impossible, but something you can hone into of the muscle group. Flex your bicep but channel from one end of the bicep to the other instead of flexing with the whole arm, so channel with a single muscle group, like the bicep, instead of channeling the whole arm. This is micro flexing.

Spells: Stream mind focus- Find your Zen pose, which is the mind's mental focus point. Use the brain frequency, or the jaw channel technique while in a focused mindset.

Steam charge- Channel from the feet to the head. Tighten and release then stream like with the advanced micro flexing above. When you get to the throat, channel up on the throat and allow your vocals to stream upwards. This does require yelling with the channel.

Ambush- Attack with multiple bursts from one arm to another. Pump one arm with advanced micro flexing, then push through the whole arm, then use the other hand. Pump channel through while alternating arms, as quickly as possible.

Advanced: To create a good o stream, stand in the 192-pointed star. Then channel, like in pathway maker on the o, up with the natural movement of the 192-pointed stars. Once you are familiar with this movement you shouldn't need to use it again.

Thunder Style

Overview: uses layers and pushes outwards

Technique: biofield manipulation, Ki connections

Knowledge: We are an electrical system. To tap into this system, we must understand the body. The nerve connects to the skin, we can feel our entire epidermis. Nerve grounds to the bone, the charge allowing the growth of blood only because of the combination of blood flowing with and against the nerve connection. With this style, we are flexing our nerves. It is important to charge the nerves before attempting this, like sitting and meditating in the sun and cross-streaming to build a charge. Next, when you flex, flex your sensation outwards, this focuses on nerve skin. Flex inwards towards the bone while concentrating on the feeling of the bone. This is nerve and bone; this will access your charge. Then flex up towards the head, while sensing your heartbeat, you should feel an excess charge from the blood and nerve combo. Now practice doing this all together.

Spells: Thunderclap- Channel through both hands and then clap. Using a micro-movement can be used with this to generate an echoed clap, which is caused by creating more movement to movement. This causes redundancy, and intensity due to an extra layer moving.

Thunder charge- Push outwards on your body. Use your nerve bone connection in the arms to push outwards on the body. Make sure you push from the inner self outwards.

Holding thunder- Hold the thundering charge and throw some punches. You will notice an increase in your punch's energy.

Thunder mode- Push out on your nerve skin connection with your nerve bone connection. Make them clash together outwards to charge even further.

Advanced: To conjure thunder, use this with conjuring, and push the sound outwards along the body to increase thunder movement.

Pressure Style

Overview: pulling from the outside in to release pressure

Technique: biofield manipulation, chi building

Knowledge: Creating qi

Qi is generated by the nerve and digestive combo, focusing on your core. These pulls of energy are easily accessible however located mostly in the core. Creating a charge with qi requires a heavy breathing technique. Moving the qi can be done with implosion channeling. With the implosion, you will naturally create a burst of energy outward once in a chi-positive state. You won't focus on the outward since it is a byproduct of implosion.

Spells: Qi pulls- Put your two fingers on your forehead. breathe in through the nose only. Pull inwards from the core and concentrate only on your fingers. Draw the power to your fingers.

The squeeze- Pull inwards with full body. Use the Qi pull while squeezing qi inwards. This will put you in a qi charge state.

Tightened focus- Channel your focused qi into a tightened one on your palm, then release. Push through with the pressure you just build up. This is a qi release.

Advanced: Use heavy concentration breathing while fighting to prolong this state. This is a way to quickly build up qi, try to absorb as much qi as possible before using your qi.

Chi blocking-

These are styles that mimic marmaluka, an old dead martial art that targets the chi points. If you know your anatomy, these arts are lethal. Know your chakra points and your anatomy and use the information holder to remember your anatomy. This is a kinesiology look at performing chi blocks, which can cause electrical patterns in the body to redirect, disrupt, or damage the nerve. These attacks combine with mixed martial styles and go well with acupuncture understanding. However, these styles can be lethal without striking vital spots. It is important to treat this with respect, or it will bite you, like playing with fire or electricity, always be careful.

Bear Style

Overview: Power of restraint

Technique: biofield manipulation, Pathway creation

Knowledge: Eye for an eye

To make yourself a machine you must exercise pain. To strike your opponent as hard as you can means you strike yourself harder. Using the bo staff can be used to toughen nerves, for example using it in a box strike, from one armpit to above shoulder, to the other armpit to shoulder, this is a simple box technique, that that can be used to strike the armpit and traps for blow striking. Using a bo staff naturally strengthens your resistance to taking a hit, using it at full strengthening and intentionally hitting yourself as hard as you can, gives maximum output for pain tolerance. When making yourself a machine, it is important to recognize the appropriate moment to fight, or not to fight. This should be executed quickly to stop or start a fight. Just because you can perform at a lethal level does not mean you should. However, it doesn't hurt to practice at that level and be prepared for anything.

Spells: bear strike- Strike while pulling back on the skin and muscles, making them channel towards the body. This holds back the strike in energy only, giving it a powerful after-hit.

Bear pump- Pump your full body with the Kaioken technique. Use bear strike while in this state.

Bear heal- Flex and pump it off, remember when you use these techniques there is a muscle cooldown. After use, the cooldown is less intense. The cooldown becomes less and less the more you use these techniques.

Advanced: You can use this style with other styles, especially any Berserker style.

Viper Style

Overview: vicious strikes leave venomous wounds

Technique: Micro sensory, Pathway creation

Knowledge: Disclaimer

It is important to understand how to heal someone as it is to not harm people. These strikes are vicious, and when you are participating with someone, they should know what you are using. Always warn participants or attackers. With participants, try to teach them as well, it's rude to hold back vital information for their growth as well. Remember this isn't about belief, it will not stop your body from performing, if they have mental blocks they should not participate, due to lack of knowledge. It is good to practice on the self-first, to practice both extraction and injection.

Spells: Venom touch- Take your finger and feel a point of it, then feel another point, then feel as many spots on your finger as possible. Push out on all those points at once to generate the venom touch.

Twisting viper- Twist the channel in your fist and forearm. Then add a twist to the strike, this causes two redundant systems, both the arm physically moving and the channel twisting at the same time.

Venom extract- Understand your magnetism and the feeling of your magnetism after the strike. Pull on the magnetism to extract your touch from the one strike. Simply by feeling the differentials between the target and you, you can heal anything you afflict.

Slither- When you touch the target, pull on the venom to draw out the touch, by pulling back on the magnetism and moving your hand in an s-like motion.

Advanced: These mixes well with mixed martial arts as well as acupuncture information.

Mantis Style

Overview: focuses on prepared strikes

Technique: Micro sensory, Pathway creation

Knowledge: Restraint

Knowing where to place your strikes is knowing acupuncture and knowing the spots for the attack. It's good to understand meridians, and other points of interest when attacking however it is not crucial to all of them. Know that you can do damage when hitting nerve bundles however not necessary with this style. This style focuses on chi blocking which can be stopped anywhere you hit, however retrieving an attack is difficult in more vital places.

Spells: Mantis strike- Pull in on your skin and channel through the pull. This is a proper chi strike.

Mantis retrieves- strike the same points that you struck and pull on the differential of the magnetism same as using venom extract. With this one, you can zip it out quickly.

Mantis claw- Pull in on your skin and channel through the bone, pushing out on your knuckles. You should get a claw effect. When using this, you will strike deeper, it is good to have restraint. This is harder to heal, you have to pull from the back and front outwards to heal.

Advanced: Greatly more effective if used with knowledge of acupuncture, as well as MMA. Please use all chi- blocking styles responsibly.

Genjutsu-

This style of fighting attacks the target's attention. These styles vary from overwhelming the opponent with feelings, to redirecting attention, or just piercing through their focus.

Enlightened Style

Overview: strikes with enlightenment

Technique: Meditation process, Emotional control

Knowledge: Enlightenment

This art is a defensive tactic for nonlethal confrontation. This art also requires enlightenment to perform, along with the ability to manifest a feeling. Understand that enlightenment can take years of practice, however, it is good to acknowledge that a path well forged can be followed swiftly. Make a foot trail into a road and it is easier to follow. This means that some practitioners may be able to get enlightenment within weeks or days. Understand that enlightenment is a physical pathway, no matter how bad or good you are, the only requirement for enlightenment is that you have a body. It is free for everyone, but the value is much deeper.

Spells: Overwhelm- Tap into enlightenment by focusing while in a Zen pose. Call upon your enlightenment and put your palm on another's forehead.

Epiphany- Epiphany is three levels deep, or three levels higher however affects you 3 layers deep. If you ever gain epiphany, strike your opponent with that feeling.

Quivering palm- Push on the presence of the being, pushing outwards on the palm. Tap into enlightenment and push outwards on the palm, you will find this has a ripple effect, it is effective vs malpractices, monsters, and the possessed. Striking the target with your palm causes the ripple within them, clearing the negative.

Advanced: This technique is to avoid battle, or to cleanse the target.

Counter Style

Overview: redirection and distraction of your opponents with the mind

Technique: boundary understanding, Third eye evolution

Knowledge: Manipulation

The key to using this style is to implicate movement away from close combat. This is a starting method, when you strike you strike the aura of the being or manipulate the aura of the being. The aura is not the being however made from. You can plant subliminal messages within your attack by maneuvering their biomagnetism by pushing on their field. You can push on them before you even get to them, and use wavelengths to cause sleeplessness, alertness, fear, or even enlightenment. You can also use this in combat up close focusing on certain body patterns, or even while escaping. This is best used with martial arts.

Spells: Sleep/awake spiral- Move both hands in an inwards spiral to cause sleepiness, the closer the more effective. Those of you with sleep trouble can massage the forehead in an inwards spiral to cause sleepiness. To cause alertness to use the outward spiral on the target and is more effective up close. However, while using the unenlightened quivering palm you can push on the enemy from a distance to cause either effect.

Redirect- Push outwards on the palm and push on the target. You can sense the vibes of the target; you can send these vibes elsewhere with a swipe. This should distract the target.

Refocus- You can also push on their vibes and throw them back at them. This may cause the target to disorientate. The more you use these techniques the more you will start to see. Read their vibes to read their mind.

Advanced: They mix well with any martial style.

Disruptor Style

Overview: destroying focus of the enemy

Technique: boundary understanding, Hidden techniques

Knowledge: Creating cracks

This style pierces through the wavelengths of the opponent. This ignores the body's wants and needs, which is part of the psychological thinking process. The left side is imagination and the right the truth, so the left also wants or creates, whereas the right is need and information. When using this technique, striking the left can disrupt their next attack, whereas the right will penetrate the defense.

Spells: Listening hand mind strike- This requires a neutral focus. Then strike with a listening hand at the target's focus spots to disrupt the form of thinking. This would be the mental flow map of the mind, striking around their side and their head.

Discharge- Create a charge in the forearm and cross the forearm with the other arm. Doing this causes a discharge of energy. build up the energy in the arm to discharge it. This can block the enemy from targeting you with an anger focus, or even other styles of genjutsu.

Puncture- Strike while using a listening hand on the focus of the foe. You can break the focus and the wavelengths the foe puts out. For these attacks, you can strike the body, and still disrupt focus. If your mind's eye can see the focus, then attack the focus of the enemy with a puncture strike.

Advanced: This goes well with mixed martial arts, however, requires training to truly utilize these techniques.

Spiritual

This is to understand what resides in the spiritual world, and how to cleanse, see, dispel, and read spirits. The spiritual realm is created by the leftovers of us. Technically a ghost should not be able to think due to lack of matter, it should not produce thought, nor can it hold thought anymore because the brain is dead. However, the recording of the moment is left over. Our singularities cause us to contrast with the singularity of the earth. Therefore, we are recorded within this singularity, in the space, we are given. Remember we only take up so much space, therefore same with a ghost. A lot of times houses are disconnected from nature, allowing spaces to be haunted instead of recycling these moments of extreme emotion. Our thoughts of darkness also cause us to have powerful singularity moments, especially in moments of fear, hate, and of course the sinister. Not everything in the spiritual is evil, just mostly what we catch that affects humans is sinister, the good doesn't bother us unless, of course, they are the greater good. It is important to understand they are dead, and no longer influence the living. Their time ended, regardless of how short it was, it is important to allow the dead to move on. Most of what you will find in the spiritual is leftovers that the earth has rejected because of their malice.

Residence-

It's important to understand what resides in the spiritual, but like a wild animal, you must find it, they are not always there. The bite of an animal cannot hurt you if it's not there, the touch of a ghost cannot hurt if it is not there. That is why we have hauntings; they are in the spot of the haunting that's all. The natural resistance of the spiritual is not human, but rather pieces of life, of that which has lived, which for longer than us, was not human. We have the flora and the fauna, which give off Mushi, with the earth as its stage, and the ancient elementals/devils.

Tender

Overview: gains the knowledge of dealing with the dead

Technique: Third eye evolution, Cleansing shi

Knowledge: Wisps

The Mushi is the Japanese understanding of the spirits. They are neither flora nor fauna, rather the leftovers of life and death in every form it may come in, including plants and animals. A tree is a common tool of the spiritual, usually sucking up souls, and releasing them into a more refined form, a form of Mushi known as wisps. Wisps are usually made of leftover emotion. When done properly we can skip the ghosts and see them recycled as wisps. Wisps come in two colors black and white, however when observed can give off their true color or what's inside. Wisps can be absorbed as well giving negative or positive chi. The best way to attract wisps is through a fairy fountain, which is using light with the 192-pointed star, causing an energy font that attracts the spiritual. Don't be afraid to use your tools.

Spells: Differentials- It's good to understand the difference between you and the things around you, especially spirits. Respect the spirits and gain respect in return.

Attracting spirits- Use the 192-pointed star with light, sound, or both to create an energy pool that will attract spirits.

Tuning- Using thermal imaging, you can capture the activity of spirits on camera around the font.

Advanced: Animals leave ghosts as well, same with trees and plants. but like animals, ghosts are only in the location they are found. Location is everything when looking for an activity. Mushi are as variant as life on earth.

Keepers

Overview: Preparing your spiritual spaces

Technique: Cleansing shi, Third eye evolution

Knowledge: Creating spaces

It is important to cleanse your space energy-wise. A house is a built environment. Knowing how a house is built can help you create a spiritual environment. First, it is good to know where the wind blows, on what side of the house, also where the sunshine is, and of course tree proximity. Where the wind blows are the most likely place where ley lines are located. Sunshine is important for many things, mostly that the energy that the sun carves into the atmosphere also creates ley lines or ray lines. Plant location is important for connecting the house further with nature. Trees near a house can be used to reconnect with nature. Conduits built in walls create the most energy in a house (conduit is used to hold electrical wires), when the conduits line up with the wind or sun it creates an energy that is aligned with the rest of the energy of the earth. Find conduits near lights or sockets that are on the windy part of the house, to establish ley lines in the house. To cleanse them there are various techniques to use, and various techniques to protect your space, and invite nature back into this separated environment.

Spells: blue fire cleansing- You can use many products, however for a slow blue flame you can use axe spray. Light the axe in a shot glass to get a flame that penetrates the spiritual. A propane torch works for cleansing ley lines or lines of energy in the house.

Dream catcher placements- Where you dream is where you'll need dream catchers. This will capture bad or good wisps. When the dream catcher gets full it becomes more aggressive. Use the blue flame to cleanse dream catchers. Letting the dream catcher get full create manifestations of a like feeling, building Oni spirits and other types of manifestations.

Attuning to space- Use a slow blue flame to attune to the space. Meditate when using this and step into the spiritual while using a blue flame. This is intimidating to other things that may exist.

Advanced: Keepers are meant for keeping a positive environment in space. Using energy scrubbers is another form of cleansing that can be used, as well as singing bowls, that can cleanse an area with their pitches. Choose the pitch that suits you to help attune the space to you.

Summoners

Overview: servants of the devil themselves

Technique: third eye training, spiritual tunning

Knowledge: Devils

Planes are specific movements of energy, that for some reason the elementals reside in. These beings are greater than us, due to existing despite not being alive. Dragons are usually protectors of the natural planes. For example, the rotation of the core creates friction creating an electrical plane, while the core itself pulls inward creating another plane while pushing outwards creating another plane. There are many other planes, however, the best way to access these is the dream. It is important to recognize something beyond yourself. The best way to access the planes is to have an octagon to invite all 8 elements. Next use crystals attuned to each element or use a piece of each element, and to further connect add a source of energy, like light or electricity to the center of the octagon. Using the third eye and or thermal imaging camera you can see if anything wishes to visit you. If one element seems stronger to you than the rest, then use all eight corners with that element to access the elementals/devils.

Spells: Symbols and devils- Elemental devils tend to be in the form of Cherubim. Cherubim include but are not limited to dragons, griffins, and or other types of beings that are pieces of other life. Humans are a form of Cherubim. When using the ritual before using a specific element invite all to the summoning and your chances of seeing one increase. Use your third eye to see the spirits. To do this you need your eyes closed and in a meditative pose.

Gifts and demeanor- Always approach with respect, never label a spirit, and allow it to make itself known. Gifts are passive, if you go in expecting nothing, you'll be surprised by what you receive. Your presence alone is a gift to the elementals; however, a gift of magic understanding is always a possibility if you can listen to what they have to offer.

Given power- Power comes from knowledge. Understand the difference between you and the power you feel from another source. This will let you receive a gift, sometimes in the form of a familiar.

Advanced: She delves into the plane of fire, and he is in the plane of thunder. These are the dragons, one with his mouth open, and the other with her mouth closed. The one eye in the void, or the wolf in the trees, the pink mothers of the universe, or the blue giants, regardless of what devil or mega spirit you encounter, if you are good and true, they may see you and you may not have to fear them. Always be cautious. Some spirits are strong enough to physically manifest into the physical, usually in black and white. These are living memories. Remember if you do get visited by a living memory it will always appear in front of you, not in your peripheral. If you gain a familiar as a gift, allow it to be itself and to do what it needs to do.

Directors-

These styles are different ways to interact with other entities, however, unlike the Mushi and the elementals, these styles deal with hauntings and more human problems, and are less nature based.

Exorcist

Overview: understanding ghosts

Technique: Cleansing shi, the Meditation process

Knowledge: Ghosts

You don't see wild animals unless you are within their territory, ghosts are the same. However, ghosts don't have a source of energy to produce themselves, this is said again for a reason. Think of it as more of a carving within layers of the magnetic sphere. Our singularities spike when we have emotional turmoil, therefore leaving a mark on our existence when we are in a heightened state before death. The release is extreme as well when our energies turn to nothing. Ghosts cannot think but are however a product of something that could. Demons have no physical, they are conjured by using a physical body or a plane. Monsters, however, have physical bodies, you should practice caution when encountering monsters. However, this focus is on ghosts. When tracking ghosts be aware of pressure differentials, the difference will feel heavy. Some ghosts are active and will try to mess with you. Here are some methods when working with ghosts.

Spells: Evergreen absorbers- Place trees in hauntings to passively take them back to nature.

Heart meditation- Meditate with your heart to cleanse your body, the energy of your body is constantly cleansing, and leaving a mark on you is impossible, you are the one alive, and your body is constantly changing, and regenerating, so the mark will pass as you shed cells. Still with the heat movement of the body, should cleanse you almost instantly.

God's presence- Tuning into the greater good presence is easy if you are on that path. Evil isn't the only thing that is leftover. God's presence will always be outside of the self and is never going to try to take over you. Parasitic ghosts, or demons, tend to try to mimic you and be you, however, are not you. We are ever-changing beings, so adapt to get away from them.

Advanced: Don't be afraid of using physical tools to help ward off spirits. The truth of ghosts is their basic truth, what they were is all they can become. Understand the truth of ghosts and death to further strengthen the self.

Guides

Overview: guides to the dead

Techniques: Cleansing shi, Third eye evolution

Knowledge: Leftovers

One theory on ghosts is that it is the leftover negative energy of an individual, as the good or the soul is absorbed by the earth. This is only because of the number of negative entities left behind because of this. The energy that is left is usually malice, hatred/intolerance, greed, jealousy, betrayal, confusion, and vengeance. These are negatives a neutral does not have. This is only a theory based on what already exists, unfortunately, without a body, it shouldn't matter, without matter there is no energy. This phenomenon does not follow the law and is cleansed with knowledge of the law. Only because we are positive in the universe that every life matters and every life is chosen, is the only reason we matter even in our passing. There is no control over death, so what has left works on an instinct basis, which can gather to form manifestations, like spirits, with similar makeup in feeling. This can happen to the positive as well. There is a way to guide the spirits into the spiritual, these are the following techniques.

Spells: 3 layers- There are about three layers to the plane of spirits or the plane of death. To banish a ghost is to put them 3 layers deeper than they are. You can use the 192-pointed star to help channel three layers.

Making gateways- Using light formations you can create a gateway for ghosts to follow. The mind is usually within the clutch of gravity. So, when beings die, usually they still follow the pattern of gravity, because that's how they remembered it. Flying ghosts are beyond that our normal patterns.

Calm cleanser- Making a presence of calm and mindfulness for the dead, is the best thing you can do when guiding ghosts to the other side.

Advanced: Putting these three techniques together is the best route to help others to the other side.

Expellers

Overview: purging spirits, and people

Technique: Cleansing shi, Pathway creation

Knowledge: Illusion of language

To communicate with ghosts, it is best to use the language the ghost could speak to ease the restless soul. Regardless of the source of language, you should understand that language is an illusion. Our first language is a lack thereof, consisting of only instinct and body language, even that can vary. Language is made up, and not the original language of all beings. The original language is the reason why we need language, the language of decay and time. Our bodies respond to the lack of resources that it needs to sustain themselves. The language that created us was geometrical and chemical. Using the 192-pointed stars, one can use this base language to expel ghosts. It can also be used as a net for demons, and a mental cleanser for people.

Spells: Mind purge- Use your brain frequency with the 192-pointed stars to cleanse the mind. You can stand in it or you can meditate in it, or even just use the book to cleanse the mind by visualizing the star in your mind to cleanse it.

Full body purge- Again you may need a larger image to use the full body scan, however with the mind's eye you should be able to do a full body scan without it. Pull up with your hands and use the frequency in your hands to cause a purge.

Person purge- Anyone in trouble just needs to see the star to be cleansed, however, a full body purge can be done on someone else if you use the star. It will leave them behind, however, erase any grasp a manifestation would have. Remember this star is like a large dream catcher.

Advanced: If you use the star with the truth, it has more of an effect. Purging large areas is also possible with this rune, cleansing areas, and purifying spirits.

Readers-

There are reading rules. The first rule is never to claim anything. To protect others and other beings, we use the signs of other people as a representation of similarity, however, sometimes the journey is that being, but is not for us to say, only that that being has a relationship with another. Only claim the self. Rule two, interpret loosely. Use things like familiarity, similarity, associated with, the era of, relative to, the journey of, student of, and of course always the possibility of it. Rule three, the meaning is always based on the individual, due to their mindset and their understanding of themselves and their journey, meaning half the interpretation is theirs. Rule Four is that life is ever-changing. We are not destined or fated, and if we are it's better not to know, that stress can damage the path. Rule Five, once you open the book, you are an open book. Looking into our past lives can change us, once we do so the book is now open, and we are now on a new path that happens only occasionally. It is like walking with eyes closed, once you open them there is so much that we can change or maneuver. The book gives no power, only direction. A soul reading is deep and gets the closest to opening the book to our journeys. Palm reading is a path we are taking, and chi reading is how we have forged ourselves on the path.

Soul Reader

Overview: interpreting the soul

Technique: Third eye evolution, Hidden technique

Knowledge: Soul reading

It is possible to read people with guardians although much harder to get a deeper look due to the guardian. They need to either release their guardian or figure it out themselves before reading. When reading a person, you will find that sometimes animals appear. Remember before humans were thousands of years of giant animals, who have the capability for learning. Intelligence comes in many forms of life and was shaped differently for thousands of years before humans. One theory is it takes 8 animal lives to equal one human life. This is suggesting before we ever came to be, if there is reincarnation, we were something else along the path of life. Regardless, the past is the past, we are merely trying to gauge where we were on our path so that we may move forward knowing what we are built for. In the end, we are a byproduct of the natural ecosystem, we have a purpose, and as intelligent beings, we have even more so the responsibility to our ecosystem; we all have a place. So, while it is possible to see what animals we journeyed as, we also have made our way through humanity. Remember the numbers of animals and beings and understand we partake in life as well, we are part of those numbers, and we will not be selfish, but for some reason, some of us have existed before. It is important not to push these possibilities on people, even if you can see the entire truth, some people can't cope with this. Only look for the ones who are willing to see, they are worthy, ones who are not willing to see are not worthy but can become worthy by excepting that the truth is not always what we want, that the truth is good and evil, it is non-biased. Truth is harder to accept when we don't understand the laws of truth. The properties of truth are that it is neutral, but while it exists for the fact, we exist as a positive or it would be nothing, and nothing would be true. We are something, our truths are positive, regardless of its evil or inequality. If you do not fear the truth, it is your weapon to wield.

Spells: Reading yourself- Focus on the third eye while meditating and using the mind's eye. All things that you see in you are you, and your journey is interpreted one way or another.

Reading others- Take the volunteer's forearm, and place one hand at the elbow and the other hand at the wrist. The channel between the two and focus on the third eye. This may give you a glimpse of them.

Combined reading- Using your third eye, you can read and gauge a person and see what they are. Play off of each others read, to get more detail of the person.

Advanced: Remember to hide when reading others, using hidden techniques.

Palm Reader

Overview: reading the hands

Technique: Dream law, Third eye evolution

Knowledge: Hidden fates

When reading the palm, always remember you are on both sides of your body. You are the left and right. These are your paths, you may lean more to one than the other, but fate lies in between your hands. This is one way to hide from fate, so no fate is certain anyways, and with this knowledge know your path lies between two paths. So, reading possibility is more likely than reading fate. Knowing the possibility we has room for mistakes, shortcomings, and failures to understand. The truth lies between two different possibilities, which are your palms. You can get the knowledge from palm reading from many different sources, in this book we work on palm gem reading, from a certain possibility, which is either left or right hand.

Spells: Asking palms- You can use the gem to read the fate of your life, by using a pendulum over the palm. Usually, we ignore asking questions, however, it can be done. Use a different pendulum than your neutral reader. Dip the stone past your hand three times, and give it purpose, like how many kids will I have, when will I die, that sort of thing. Center it about an inch over your palm. Hold it still while it moves. Circles and oval movements are usually the difference between something, like yes, no, or girl, and boy. Alternate hands to see two different fates.

Self-asking- You can do this to yourself and see the difference between the two fates.

Partner asking- Using a partner to hold the gem, you can see your fate between the two fates, however, there are many fates between the two, it is unseeable, but the result can be scary when you have both hands touching, with thumbs out.

Advanced: Starting of movement, stopping of movement, pauses, and starting movement are all time variables.

Chi Reader

Overview: reading chi

Technique: Dream law, Third eye evolution

Knowledge: Fundamentals of chi

To find chi use the Zen drop technique, to see the chi further you must use your third eye. Chi will flare up in the right position. The chi will always be a resemblance of the elements. Remember the elements are everything that is something. Chi representation is like seeing the flow of the mind, and personality combined. When looking for chi you must look not at what you want to be but at what you are. If you want to change or strengthen your chi, you must be different to do so. Someone experienced might have levels of representation. The idea is we are never the same in every life, so to see chi is to see the default you in this life. Chi can be seen in different ways, one way is the inner instinctual flow of chi within you giving you your spirit, your martial chi. Martial chi is found using meditation and tai chi at the same time. Instead of flowing with movement, flow with your instinct, and see what you find. Refine your instinct to find your martial chi, by practicing your chi flow.

Spells: Proper positioning- Find your Zen pose, the pose which gives focus, and ignites your chi. For greater detail go to Zen sage.

16 personalities- Your heart is one element and the mind another, all attached to a wheel of chi types. Your personality is a combination of chi to ignite greater combos. Find what personality you are, then find what type of chi you are. Listen to the third eye with the mind's eye to see your chi.

Flowing with chi- Meditate on the center of yourself, focus on your center, and flow with your instinct. Flowing with chi means you can flow with your instinct, revealing the very nature of you whether it be dancing or fighting you can unlock your chi by listening to your core center and moving with the reaction.

Advanced: You can learn more about your chi when you flow in a mind's eye open state, and how it reacts with others.

Materialist

Materials are just that, but can be something more when put to valuable use. To understand the material value, we must understand the value of the material. Due to matter not being able to be destroyed, just reshaped, the matter of the earth is very much a set value of matter. Other than the northern lights, which are the plasma of the sun (matter) hitting our atmosphere, there is no other way to obtain more matter than the earth has, so we must be careful when shooting matter into space. Regardless, the universe is not lack matter it is full of it. We would be able to create monstrous ships the size of the earth if we had access to all the matter on Jupiter, we could create an army of earth-sized ships, and Jupiter would still have more matter to spare. The matter is abundant, and we have bountiful nature to thank for this. Eventually, we will be able to create any material from any material with advanced alchemy. Matter transforms already, learning to aid it is the next goal.

Earth-

Using items to gain healing effects, or other effects, create the whole of usage into a new realm of learning. Using gemstones, we can see the lack of or abundance of the chakras. We use the proper stones for proper effects. We use metals for their innate properties. Materials are there to aid life, not to devalue it. Use what the earth gives you, but respect what it can do for you.

Stone Mage

Overview: learn to use stones

Technique: Eternal knowledge, boundary Understanding

Knowledge: Stones

Stone comes in different forms of representation. Each stone is like an emotion, that can be held and felt differently based on its makeup. Some stones hold a flavor and react differently based on the individual. To feel stone, you must taste it with touch. Remember to do this you must understand the difference, which was based on the full feeling of the structure, versus the taste of the individual molecules that create the stone. Crystals have different properties allowing them to be used in specific ways, whereas stones have set reactions and different properties than crystals. This focus is on using stone.

Spells: Fortified stone- Use stones to fortify a feeling or an aid to your situation. Depending on the type of stone depends on the feeling it fortifies.

Stone drag- Drag the stone in your hand in the air and feel the charge of the earth drag on the stone. This is to cleanse the stone.

Feeling stone- Cleanse your hand and feel the reaction of the stone with you. Colored stones tend to have a chakra reaction.

Advanced: Dragon bloodstone is good for cleansing, whereas shugnite has dark physical reactions. Seer stones tend to have positive reactions with the third eye. Chakra stones, or colored stones, tend to tell you how your chakra type is doing, high reactions usually mean a lack of that color in your body, meaning it is a system you need to exercise. Sometimes you can feel toxicity if you exercise that color in a bad way, usually being some sort of addiction. Other times you may get a faint feeling meaning you have low reactivity to the color, and that system is usually ok. Stones follow the rule of that which needs to be healed yield a higher reaction, and a lower reaction if the system does not need healing. You can use the mind's eye technique to further see the reaction of stone with a person.

Gem Sage

Overview: uses gems for healing

Technique: Eternal knowledge, boundary understanding

Knowledge: Gems

Gemstones hold power in their growth. The way the gemstone was formed is like its birth, giving them its personality. Cutting with grains is like cutting with its established personality. Gems, unlike stone, can absorb heat and even frequencies. They can hold a charge, like glass which is similar in this perspective.

Spells: Gem charge- Putting gems out in the sun is the best way to charge the stone. You can also use lights and lamps for this. To replay the gem use a magnetic field.

Chakra amplification- You can amplify chakras with matching gems and can absorb the excess if needed. The best way to absorb is after the gem is charged.

Gem reactions- The color of the gem gives a basis for its reactions. It can tell you what needs to be strengthened and what needs to be focused, on or if it's overused.

Advanced: You can use gems in many things, to learn to carve frequencies on gems go to crafting.

Alchemist

Overview: using metals for aiding power

Technique: Eternal knowledge, Pathway creation

Knowledge: Prime of metal

As the electron surveillance orbit becomes full, the center two move in a way to create gasses. The way these works is based on the geometrical alignments becoming greater when there are more electrons. For example, carbon has four outside surveillance electrons, and nitrogen has five. The degree differential between a square and a pentagon is enough to cause movement in the inner two. That 18 degrees is enough to make carbon solid, and nitrogen gas. Numbers have their properties, multiples have properties based overall, creating their properties, whereas primes always hold the prime property. Silver, gold, and copper are all prime metals, meaning they all have specific properties related to all being primes. This property is to create electricity when magnetism is present. Metals affected by magnetism work differently with the body.

Spells: Gold cleansing- Gold naturally cleanses the plasmic space of water. Gold is good to wear, and good for cleansing the blood's charge. This makes gold good for those who have been afflicted or possessed.

Copper channeler- The balance of copper makes it so useful. Wearing copper can cause a change in the copper. When you use channeling and pinpoint channeling you can create a charge in the copper. It can also absorb heat, as well as gain a charge. Copper is great for channeling.

Silver healer- Silver has high organic reactions, and in specific solutions is good for the body. It is said silver ingested can turn the body blue, which is a connection to the Yondu in the Hindu religion where beings from another planet were blue. be careful with silver, take only what is recommended, silver has a high organic reaction, meaning wearing silver is for healing purposes.

Iron protection- Iron is known to have protective properties and is good for warding off spirits, which technically means we are spirit resistant, due to the iron in our blood. It also reacts with us, so wearing iron for protection, and its reaction to magnetism makes it work well for using the blood circulation with iron, to give it a charge.

Advanced: For further uses of metals go to crafting.

Plant

Plants are the epiphany of the bountiful earth, being a renewable resource. While they are living, they are not alive, they rely on the magnetism of the planet to create their singularity. This suggests that plants are a tool of nature. Without plants, the cycle of life stops. Plants provide food for herbivores, which is needed to sustain carnivores, where the plants go the herbivores go, and so forth. They are essential for cleaning the air and providing shelter for us when needed. Plants do so much, however, are not a true singularity. Regardless they are the most positive of life; for the most part they are all giving. Therefore, plants are a tool of life, just to sustain us. We are the result of the cycle of life. Understanding this we understand how important plants are. Trees have their properties and importance, whereas plants have different uses. Know that water and its level of cleansing changes the potency of plants and the feel of trees. How you cleanse your water is very important.

Tree Mage

Overview: understanding the power of the tree

Techniques: Cleansing shi, Eternal knowledge

Knowledge: Power of trees

Trees don't have circulatory systems; however, they do have sap that acts as a connectivity to the rest of the tree. The sap feeds off the magnetism of the earth and gives its signal. The tree uses the redundancy of the signal to layer up, meaning the rings of the tree are meant to spiral, but we see them as rings because it grows all at once. The spiral nature naturally creates rings of redundancy. We see in organic life the pattern of the spiral; trees are no different. All these properties go into using the tree. The tree is created for a positive niche. Meaning it was made literally for usage, the all-giving tree.

Spells: Layered absorption- Trees have multiple layers of absorption. You can use multiple layers of absorption like a tree. Pull in on the skin and feel the layers of absorption, all the way to the core. Organs act as layer of absorption and can absorb wavelengths. This is a defensive tactic.

Tree ground- Use a tree to ground the self out, this takes away a specific magnetism, that which isn't yours.

Tree whisperer- Observe where the tree has been or will be and understand that the tree listens. Redundancy of life conformation, that it existed and therefore it is, meaning if it existed for hundreds of years, and then was cut down, it can leave a mark of its existence. Essentially ghost trees can be seen with the third eye. Trees that live can leave auras, and some trees are so old that they have a deeper connection to the world than we do.

Advanced: Tree sap can be used to absorb a frequency, the tips of new branches, and buds, are an awesome source for wand making, and the bark of enchanted trees is useful in many ways. To make an enchanted tree, one must grasp the feelings and knowledge of the 16 elements. This is a new feeling that the trees respond to, allowing growth and teamwork. The blessing is a Vanahiem blessing, the realm of the other gods in Norse mythology. Knowledge is required for this. See eternal knowledge.

Plant Sage

Overview: usage of plants

Technique: Eternal knowledge, Third eye evolution

Knowledge: Plants

Plants are very physically literal. Their properties won't change; however, they can be reorganized. Understanding that before modern medicine we used plants in test trials on their effects on us. Using the soil as a guide to what type of plants is essential. For example, you can find a poisonous root plant by its bitter touch. You can gain a sense of what is around simply by what type of soil is naturally around. Plants use water and soil to give signals, giving what they produce, or take as a byproduct. How they function is directly related to their byproducts. Plants can also sense vibration, so they can sense our energetic bodies because of their vibration and temperature differentials. Essentially, they have the most basic form of communication, however the hardest to use within us due to their natural complexity. Here are some other outside uses for plants.

Spells: Tracing herbs- The soil leaves trace elements of plants and what they use in it. Feel the soil near known herbs and feel the difference between soil near them and away from them. You should feel the difference between enriched soil and not used soil. The difference in the feeling of soil is key to understanding the plants in an area. Take soil near a tree vs near the herb, you'll find the soil is different in texture due to the tree. The amount of water absorbed will leave a moisture difference. Poisonous root plants will leave a bitter feeling in the soil. Be careful when working with unknown plants, always use a guide when exploring new plants.

Plant healing- Using the harmony technique on plants will help the plant stabilize itself and give a new pattern that's dormant in the plant.

Teaching plants- Plants can learn, but we must be the ones to teach them. Using eternal knowledge, you can teach the plant a feeling and activate something within itself. This may reorganize the taste of food as well, giving a new and improved version of the fruit, which changes its seedlings as well.

Advanced: signals of plants can travel through water, so affecting the water can change your plant. Use positions for this.

Potions

Overview: how to make potions

Technique: Eternal knowledge, Pathway creations

Knowledge: Changing water

Cleansing water is essential to creating potions or enhancing plants. First is always the physical filter to filter physical elements out of the water. Next is to filter the plasmic space of the water using gold and glass. You can use light in different ways to cleanse water, like ultraviolet light to kill germs. This process is similar however using indirect electricity with the water to clean it based on the signal of cleansing or other words using gold. You can use silver which has a high organic reaction, for healing properties in silver different ways. Copper is used indirectly, like using light, and iron can be used indirectly as well. Here are some basic uses of water and metal.

Spells: Healing water- Never put the metal in contact with the water. Wrap the silver wire around a glass and shine a light on the glass and silver. You can use the 192-pointed star to drag the frequency through the water. This should change the water taste. You can do this in other ways; however, this is the simplest way.

Purified water- You want to use the same tactic with gold wire. This should cleanse the plasmic space and make water taste pure. The better the first filter the better results you will get.

Warding water- You want to use the same tactic with iron wire. This should make the water warding.

Advanced: Once you purify the water, you can use it for plants, brewing, and even cooking. There are many ways to get further information on positions and other things, however, the difference is the water.

Crafting

Magic would die without niches in crafting, otherwise what is the point? Remember only a physical literal pathway will arise in its greatest form. Metals already have very powerful properties, however, can be attuned to energies, such as the six energies. These energies can also be carved onto crystals and are associated with specific shapes.

Enchanter

Overview: enchanting metals

Technique: Pathway creation, Sorcery mechanics

Knowledge: Enchanting

The way you shape metal already gives it its primary intent. If you shape it to kill it will kill, if you shape it to protect, it will protect. The way you shape it is its intent, a shield is not a sword, and a sword is not a shield. Using the proper materials for their based properties, like conductivity, and heat absorption is another thing to think of when using enchanting. The power of organic intent can be channeled through metals, usually only associated with frequency. There are ways to harness the frequency of the area to get the desired effect. A combination of materials or beings is usually what creates effects.

Spells: Planting intent- First is using the correct metals with the correct representation. Planting intent helps with the correct metal setup.

Channelers- Gold copper and silver are the best metals for conductors, however not limited to just those, brass, bronze, tin, and steel also are semiconductors. Tin is best for channeling heat, however, most metals work for heat, light, and vibration. Magnetism works primarily with iron cobalt and nickel. Use these materials for the desired channeling properties.

Enchanted materials- The best way to enchant is by finding a "holy spot" one that resonates with an organic presence of holiness. Whereas most spots are not accessed, however, blessing material holds the intent of the blade. Although this is rare, planting intent can be easy on the metal. burying a metal with a charged stone, such as what follows, can give the metal a charge. You can also do this by burying a piece of metal in hallowed earth, or with enhanced soil from plants, to give a greater charge to the metal.

Advanced: Equipment is one thing, what metals to use, and such, but to further the channeling ability mix with etching.

Etcher

Overview: carving on crystals

Technique: Pathway creation, Sorcery mechanics

Knowledge: Etching

Using light, we can carry frequencies on the light. These frequencies can leave impressions of their movement on crystals and glass. This is like recording on a record player, but instead of vinyl, we use other materials to record energy. Sound leaves notches, and is harder to record, and harder to play back. If we use energy frequencies, we can carve frequencies that can be played back with a magnet. To record a frequency, you need the physical material present. Whatever you have present will be what you record. The following is the practice of etching: First you need a large magnet (old speaker works), a base, a lamp, and metal tweezers. Then you'll need quarts crystals, or glass. These are for being etched on. Next, you shine the lamp on the magnet with the crystal or glass on it. You are going to pull on the lamp light, with the tweezers, and create a connection while the tweezers are in the light. Remember we can create a connection with light. Next, use the tweezers to channel the light to the crystal. You are going to channel down the tweezers to cause the connection, and to the crystal or glass. Use the tweezers to mark the glass or crystal with light. Push through the tweezers when doing this, and open and close the tweezers to gain a connection. Make sure you wear rubber gloves to hide your frequency or use the hidden technique to hide your frequency. Do the following to put on different frequencies.

Spells: Electrical frequencies- Use a bulb with the wattage you want to mark on the glass or crystal. Using a higher-wattage bulb gives you a higher yield. Drag the electricity instead of the light to get electrical frequencies.

Light frequencies- Use the base technique of light with different colored bulbs to get different colors of light. Heat tempering- Use a flame with the crystal to condense the heat into the crystal.

Organic frequencies- Use a piece of paper under the crystal and use emotions on the paper. Paper can hold emotion.

Directional focuser- You can create grounds, focusers, and channelers by focusing the electricity in a specific fashion, depending on what you are pulling from. Knowing where your ground and neutral is good for these etches.

Advanced: These crystals or glass can be played back with magnets. This mixes well with enchanting, weaving, or techno mage.

Runic

Overview: axiom of symbols

Technique: Pathway creation, Sorcery Mechanics

Knowledge: Literal shape movement

Geometry is the language of reality. It creates itself into specific shapes, because of the properties of the circle, so the circle is the language of reality. When objects reach a specific size, they have specific properties that they have specifically because of the shape they are. The literal translation is in the property of the shape matter takes. No matter the size, the shape has meaning. Here are some literal shapes with meaning for creating telekinetic tattoos.

Spells: Three dots- Create 3 dots interconnected into an equilateral triangle. This can be placed anywhere from the palm to the third eye, it is a way of distributing energy. You can use a pen or marker to practice with these tools.

Inner wraith- The dot within the circle, the circle being dark and the dot being white or plain also gives a good point of push. Use a line to connect the dot to other runes.

Battery symbols- Use the yin and yang in a rectangle or circle to use as a battery.

Structural symbols- Triangles and ridges can be used to create pathways and can create resistance, or intensity to the inner wraith or the three dots.

Advanced: Make sure you have a good idea of what you want before you tattoo yourself. Using a pen or maker to practice what you think you want and use it to see if the pattern is valid or working. These markings are used for channeling and for spell usage.

Miscellaneous

These are advanced understandings that come with powerful techniques. They require tuning into truth, using advanced weapons, and forbidden techniques that can only be used by those who understand the good in the dark side. Truth can be tuned into using the 192-pointed star, and Deja Vu. Knowing what equipment to use is important for a wizard. Taming the dark side comes with the realization of the truth of nature. All these have advanced forms of understanding to utilize these techniques.

Truth-seekers

Creating a truthful environment is required for the following. becoming an avatar requires the spirit to come to you. However, with a specific mindset, and a cleansed mind, you can have the secrets of the greater spirits. bards tap into the understanding of the imagination to attune it to truth, or at least to find truth in it. Inquisitors use the truth to dispel major spells that are considered malpractice. Each one of these is the aspect of the greater light.

Avatar

Overview: Channeling greater spirits

Technique: Meditation process, Mindscape building

Knowledge: Responsibility for channeling

There is a system of gods or spiritual beings that exist to guide humanity in the right direction. Most of them are passive, so gaining access requires meditation. Sometimes they visit to protect individuals, but most of the time if you were meant to channel, they will appear in your life when you reach that given point for one reason or another. They can appear to give messages, they can appear to give understanding, protection, or guidance. To become an avatar is an honor, it means you fight for something more. The key to channeling spirits is opening the self-up and being open-minded. Be ready for an answer, and be ready and willing to submit yourself to another. Understand they cannot control you; you must allow them to control you to truly channel them.

Spells: Allowing control- When you are receiving a direct message from them, allow your body to be an instrument for the greater benevolent ghost. Usually, they give answers so wait for the answers to gain answers. You can call upon them once they have interacted with you, using a manifestation of the memory gives a direct line to the greater benevolent spirit once contact has been made.

Understanding goals- Understand that a greater spirit always comes with goals for the betterment of humanity and life. Sometimes they come in times of protection, or times of endangerment, however, must wait until you are ready to further your understanding, or have achieved an understanding that aligns with the goals of the spirit. being an avatar is also being a messenger. If you want nothing to do with it, then don't try this. be ready to spread their message.

Using powers- Some greater benevolent spirits come with ways to defend themselves. Listen to your body to mimic its power. Remember the system of gods usually forms beings that once existed.

Advanced: This, is an advanced style and technique that can take years before this happens to you. Remember to keep an open-mindedness when attempting higher communication.

Bard

Overview: Tuning into the past

Technique: Meditation process, Dream law

Knowledge: Organizing information

Sometimes when stories are told they fall into being retold stories of the past, or even from distant pasts, such as stories somewhere else in the universe. Imagination can allow a glimpse into the past, or even the future if you understand ways to pick it out. One way is to understand possibility. The closer it is to a real situation the closer it is to the truth. This is a possibility transforming into a probability. With enough detail and scientific reality, we get more of the truth. Know that possibility can come into play, usually through multiple imaginations that hang on a topic and can appear in an ⅔ ⅓ pattern. The first two will always look similar, and the ⅓ will be similar but from a very different source. For example, the Norse and the Celtic have similar seeds of life and are connected by the information being so close sources of each other, whereas the Chinese also have a seed of life like the others without connected sources. Here are some ways to sense the truth.

Spells: Feeling the truth- Using the 192-pointed star, whisper a truth onto it. The feeling that responds is usually a dark reality, but cleansed and truthful. It will feel like a Deja Vu. Using the truth is harder than detecting it, once you detect the truth you can feel that truth, however, to get there sometimes you need a truth that is a scientific solid.

Truth in a story- Stories aren't always truthful, but sometimes they retain a truth within them. Thousands of stories have happened over time, and many of them repeat or have the same elements as a previous story. Sometimes they get stuck in a loop when telling the story due to the strength of the story due to it being retold. These stories will resonate with truth. The strength of the resonance is simply the truth. Once you can sense truth, you can sense this resonance of truth in old stories.

Singling out the truth- Using the star you can single out the truth in the story. To be a bard is to single out historical truth, and retell it in a fancy fashion, like adding a little makeup to the truth. However, sometimes the truth is dark and not what we want. It is important to know that darkness is also part of reality. To be a bard you must be neutral to see the whole story.

Advanced: You can use this in other stories to pick out the truth. Use the patterns to find deeper meaning in stories as well, or to find something that might have a truth.

Inquisitor

Overview: Defense against the dark arts

Technique: Dream Law, Eternal Knowledge

Knowledge: Logic

Logic is sometimes the greatest weapon against malpractices. One of the most common mistakes is to say we have a soul that can leave the body. We are a chemical differential at 98 degrees, they are simply taking heat, the soul is an intangible idea and is not part of the anatomy. If it is it is generated by the body like the mind. This idea that we are just matter is the most physical literal, which protects us from vampirism and soul thieves. The body cannot evolve outside of its parameters unless otherwise using genetic coding to become something else, it is impossible unless of course we shape ourselves differently, however, to retain that shape requires the right code. So wereism is a not possible without the physically chemical code. Wishes can be selfish, but to get anything in life you must do it, so a wish breaks laws to give what it wants, the wish is also a not a possibility. There is too much extra to create any of these things, and too long have others feed off the ignorance of others to gain an advantage over others.

Spells: Quantum axiom- When something puts out an incorrect vibe or a violent vibe, to check it ask for its quantum axiom, its self-evident proof that at the molecular level they can produce that, from fictional pleasure vibes to malice xenomorph, ask the creature for the truth of its structure, not its energy. This is energy check- based knowledge.

Mushify- Holding power or a curse, a feeling of ailment that is not created by the self, can be held in a moment of time. This will transform the thought into a Mushi, a moment in time. To do this you need to target the feeling and release the feeling. This will clear away what is not supposed to be in time. You can also do this to people, to push on an affliction and use the realization of the feeling to pull it off. Using differentials, we can target these moments and pull it away.

Wrath of knowledge- Find a truth of why something is in malpractice and hold to that feeling. Use that feeling in your aura, channel it into a weapon, or channel out the hand with that feeling of that truth. Use your knowledge as weapon against malpractice.

Advanced: To gain more, study how things are just not possible and know that if technology can do it, then that is the truth of how it is done. This is a way to stop malpractice and afflictions. Afflictions can be destroyed, and dispelled, or pulled off, by understanding the differentials of the source and yourself.

Battlemages-

Battlemages use items to empower themselves. Taking items into the dream is one way to protect themselves, using wand combos to weave frequencies, and using technology to push further power past ourselves. Each uses items in different ways to battle, or to protect themselves from the physical, or the dream.

Spirit Warrior

Overview: warriors of the dream and spiritual

Technique: Meditation process, Dream law

Knowledge: be prepared

When creating an enhanced weapon, it is good to give it purpose or intent for taking it with you. Meditating in a circle or octagon is great for reaching the dream, however, the best way is laying down in an octagon or circle and being ready to sleep in that area. Remember to sleep with the wand or weapon sheathed. Practice safely and you can practice longer. Choosing the right tool depends on your purpose, whether for war, peace, protection, understanding, or any other reason should line up with the metal you take with you, the items you prepare, or even what you are wearing. This is how you use it.

Spells: Weapon sleep- This requires a charged weapon, make sure you have it sheathed when sleeping with a weapon, to not hurt yourself. Wands are good to bring with you to sleep. Use full body sleep with a hand grabbing onto the weapon. During sleep, you can conjure the power of the weapon by feeling the weapon in your hand.

Summoning weapon- become familiar with your crafted enchanted equipment. As you do, you may be able to summon your equipment in the dream. To do this all you need is to think about that item and pull it towards you or think of the summon coming to you, or out of the ground, or just magically appearing depending on what feeling you can conjure in thought.

Recalling weapon- If the weapon is stolen from you in the dream, if it is a physical item in your possession, then you should be able to summon it right back, especially if you are sleeping with it, or if you simply think of your possession over it. Don't get attached to spirit weapons or abilities that you can do in the dream, however, if it has reactions in the dream realms it may be valid. If you stick with reality, they can't change it or remove it.

Advanced: To recall yourself in the dream to wake up, feel the whole of yourself to force yourself awake. Try not to be violent in the dream, but everything dreams, including animals, and monsters, so be wary of their presence.

Weaver

Overview: manipulator of wavelengths

Technique: Pathway creation, Qi connections

Knowledge: Wand making

You need a thick enough stick to drill a hole in, or you can use a metal pipe, however, how you use it can differ depending on the choice. Next, you put in a magnet, this can vary from malachite pieces to high-powered neodymium magnets. Next, you put in a filler which can range from carved crystal, a colored crystal, or even copper wire. If the magnet is first and the filler second, you are on the right track. The secret to a wand is the battery. You can use actual batteries, however in the most basic cause use plants, from evergreen tips to a potato. This can vary however gains the best energy with a growing part of the plant. Using crystals with frequencies carved on to them should be the last or first thing you use depending on the pattern imprinted on the crystal. Wands can vary in how you want to make them, know that when you are creating your wand you can use personal frequencies for your wand.

Spells: Using wands- Wands are simple to use. All you need to know is to channel energy. Channel that energy through an item, and the item naturally acts as a pathway. Push through the item. This will give it the power it needs for a push. Switch around the objects in the wand if you feel like finding your fit of use.

Connecting to wavelength- Start by using the wand with light. Push on the light, or with the light to give the light your wavelength. When connected you can choose to focus further and intensify the light or add the frequency of the wand to the light. You can connect to radio wavelengths, blueTooth, and even high energy frequency. Remember the stronger the frequency the harder it is to manipulate the frequency. You can also use this with trees, electricity, and metal.

Adding to the wand- You can strengthen your wand with magnifying glasses, like from old telescopes, or you can create tips and hilts for the wand adding other frequencies. Don't add too many frequencies or they'll overlap or subdue each other.

Advanced: Making wands on their own is a whole variety of patterns and already an advanced technique. Please feel free to create more patterns with wands.

Techno Mage

Overview: magic and technology combined

Technique: Pathway creation, Sorcery mechanics

Knowledge: batteries work with a push; they have a small metal tack in the back that pushes through the battery. When we use batteries, make sure that the positive face is pointed up. With these we can push through flashlights, causing them to brighten, you can also use tasers to do the same thing, which pushes outward. Using a taser with a metal body works best. Make sure you use protection when performing with anything with a battery. Rubber gloves, electrical tape, and other insulated items help against electricity.

Spells: Taser push- Make sure you have a metal taser for the most effective push. Use an insulated glove when playing with a taser. Channel through the battery of the taser to get an effective arc. This will use up the battery quicker, so finding a metal taser with replacement batteries is the best fit. Always point downwards for the arc fans out.

Taser flood- You can flood a room with electricity if you use the taser with both hands to channel. be aware of your surroundings.

Light flood- You can also do this with metal flashlights. With light, you can redirect the electricity to travel on the light by pushing through the battery. by pulling in on the battery you can pull in on heat, or even sound.

Advanced: Using any form of berserker works well with this. Using any kind of movement or any distribute style is also advisable.

Forbidden-

These techniques are considered taboo. However, when use properly with proper understanding, these techniques are more probable and stronger. Learn to bind spirits to your whim, how to cause curses, or even to use the dark side to your advantage.

Warlock

Overview: binding of spirits

Technique: Sorcery mechanics, Cleansing shi

Knowledge: The Mushi trap

Using the 192-pointed star allows for the making of an energy font that can be used for attracting Mushi. Welling energy on the star is what causes the attraction. Having an enchanting station with this can be used to carve the Mushi to a crystal, binding it to the crystal. This is the bases of creating summons. The more physically present the summon the more powerful the carving will be. Just because it has the frequency doesn't mean it is it, it is a copy of a frequency. So you aren't really taking the spirit, you are coping the frequency of the spirit.

Spells: bait carving- This carving is to get a stronger spirit. First, you have the enchanting setup in the middle of the 192-pointed stars. Then you use different colored light to attract wisps. You can also carve the crystal with grass to attract specific types of Mushi.

Dark Mushi- To attract a minor wisp, place a dream catcher in the middle of the 192-pointed stars with the bait carving in the middle. Next wait for a dark Mushi to journey to the center of the star. You should trap it and be able to carve its feeling onto a crystal.

Playing back Mushi- Once it's carved you can use the crystal by channeling through the crystal or using a magnet. This will allow it to show its true form. You are now its master. It will play through you based on its aspects, like wraith, fury, hunger, anger, and even other aspects based on the nature of its origin. Remember it is a copy of what you capture.

Advanced: Remember carving a frequency is like a copy of what it was, you don't have to have the Mushi on you to do it. You can also carve feelings of enlightenment, God touches, and other types of positive feelings by using the ability to manifest a feeling. Use paper to capture the feeling and manifest the feeling while etching. The choice is yours to make and does not make it worse, either way, it's how you use it which makes it bad.

Voodoo

Overview: frequency manipulator

Technique: Sorcery mechanics, Pathway creation

Knowledge: Strongest voodoo

Voodoo is only as strong as the feeling, which means it's just a feeling. However, to make a feeling linger requires the practice of placing an object in the vicinity of the target. To do this yarn or paper is used to hold biological frequencies. The best way to be more effective is to carve the frequencies on crystals and playback the frequencies with magnets. Here are some ways of doing this.

Spells: Love and hate- You can carve love, although it is a reaction of two people. You can carve the feeling of your love on the crystal. You can also carve an in-general love on the crystal. You can also do this with hate, and other dark feelings, especially if they're focused on a target.

Voodoo grenade- To play this back you need to stuff a pipe with a magnet and a crystal, with dirt or sap to charge the crystal, then bury it in the location of the target to cause it to do what you want. You can also add yarn or paper to help hold the organic feeling.

Side effects- Manipulating individuals is considered the dark side, so placing the crystal to manipulate passively aggressively is the most effective way. Once you start messing with people physically, there is always repercussion, this is to avoid that.

Advanced: This is a dark practice; however, this is the best way to do this to make it real, without dealing with spirits or dark contracts, which are false anyways. Always be self-reliant. The most physical literal way is the strongest way always. Superstition usually doesn't follow science, so the fear of superstition is simply worry. Don't let worry dictate your life.

Sith

Overview: Control of the dark side

Technique: Chi charging, Emotional control

Knowledge: Hatred

The dark side is neutral, when used by some that don't understand this, it becomes chaotic and uncontrollable. Feelings are the bases of our natures, so to control the dark side one must have a neutral stance. Anger comes with focus, and to do this we must direct ourselves to a target to focus our anger on the target. Hate can work the same way, if we use a vague and general hatred for something, we can direct it to another. The difference between anger and hate is intensity. Here are some ways to harness the power of anger.

Spells: Seething- Focus your chi by breathing in and out through the nose. Focus on something that you hate, like intolerance, subjugation, enslavement, selfishness, neglect, or even purposefully ignorant. Focus on what makes you mad and use the breathing technique to strengthen your dark chi.

Anger focus- Use anger as done in Emomancer and call upon anger. You can help manifest true anger with one of the seething suggestions. Anger causes focus, so focus on an object to refocus your anger on people. You can pinpoint your anger focus by choosing what to focus on, like an arm or a leg, or even the object you wield.

Hate in general- You can use hate using the seething suggestions and use one of the Berserker techniques to channel your hatred. If you focus on the big picture, you should be able to access the hate, you could even make your hatred stronger when it is at a personal level. To hate all things with no reason is the fallen Sith. Always focus on a target and use a neutral base to allow the call upon and cool down aspects of it.

Advanced: If you succeed in holding hate, then you should also practice holding the general principles of love, by thinking of good things, like kindness, not usually directed to an individual but in general. The true evil of the Sith is in selfishness. These properties can be wielded by the righteous, so it is all about how you use it. Don't be a fallen Sith.

These techniques mix and match further the more you study. These following pages are for your creativity, to make every book not the same with further spells, and further knowledge to every book to make this spell book yours as much as possible.

Your additions:

About The Author

I am a HVAC technician for 10 years, studied in the way of refrigeration, combustion, electricity, and plumbing. I found myself on a spiritual journey that has taken me 7 years to develop a range of techniques for enlightenment. I self-studied the universe, using available resources to study a range from quantum physics, to tachyon theory, to explain the possibility of magic. This is the end result of that journey.

www.ingramcontent.com/pod-product-compliance
Lightning Source LLC
Chambersburg PA
CBHW040141110726
48005CB00018B/2600